New Zealand's Worst Disasters

True Stories That Rocked A Nation

Graham Hutchins
Russell Young

16
EasyRead Large

RHYW

Copyright Page from the Original Book

First published 2015

Exisle Publishing Limited,
P.O. Box 60-490, Titirangi, Auckland 0642, New Zealand.
'Moonrising', Narone Creek Road, Wollombi, NSW 2325, Australia.
www.exislepublishing.com

A catalogue record for this book is available from
the National Library of New Zealand.

ISBN 978-1-77559-203-7
ePub ISBN 978-1-77559-249-5

Text design and production by IslandBridge
Cover design by Nick Turzynski, redinc
Incidental illustrations from shutterstock.com
Map by Fran Whild

TABLE OF CONTENTS

Introduction

During the course of the past 160 years New Zealand has experienced many disasters, some major, some less so. A number of them are distinctive and rooted in the very character of the country. They have become part of our heritage, and in learning about them we get a glimpse of New Zealand's social history as the country evolved into a modern democracy.

Over the years memory dims. The human mind has a propensity for wiping out unpleasant memories. As a result, some disasters have receded down the memory tracks of those who were there or survived them. Not all details are handed down, verbally or in written form. Some remain just hazy recollections. For this reason we felt it important to revive accounts of long-ago tragedies and to acquaint readers with events of which they may not be aware. Out of learning about such adversity we can see how ordinary Kiwis have been able to react positively. As well as the innocent becoming victims, the ordinary can also become heroes. Our short history is peppered with such human transformations. We hope that the lessons learned in earlier disasters will continue to be applied when, inevitably, disaster descends on us again.

Major disasters like the Napier earthquake, the Erebus air accident, the Tangiwai rail disaster and the sinking of the *Wahine* are not hazy recollections. They remain very much in the public consciousness, often because of the heavy loss of life.

Most New Zealanders can recall where they were and what they were doing when the devastating Christchurch earthquake hit in 2011. It reminded us that disasters can strike with a sudden randomness that destroys our confidence in safety factors installed to prevent or limit the damage caused by such upheavals. Yet Christchurch was not our largest recorded quake. In 1855, a much bigger earthquake shook the southern regions of the North Island and the northern reaches of the South Island. Property damage was serious but very few people lost their lives.

New Zealanders displayed early on a willingness to adapt to their natural environment as best they could. Wild weather and flooding were always going to present challenges. On land, storm systems led to uncommon levels of rainfall which in turn swelled rivers and streams which often broke their banks. Death by drowning was so common here that it became known as 'the New Zealand death'.

Both on land and at sea New Zealanders would be at the mercy of the elements in days when sophisticated weather forecasting was not available. But even in more recent times we could be caught out. The demise of the *Wahine* occurred in freakish circumstances when two storm systems combined to produce conditions that were unique.

So with the best will in the world, even in a country as supposedly benign as New Zealand, things will go wrong, unusual sets of variables will come into play, Mother Nature will show no mercy and significant disasters will involve or confront us.

As the new country developed its infrastructure, with roads, railways, bridges and larger, safer shipping, it wasn't just the forces of nature that tripped us up. Human error became a factor in either causing the calamity or in not heeding warnings provided by cues of nature. Serious fires and transport accidents often fell into this category.

There were several rail disasters in the years when train travel was a dominant means of getting around. The Tangiwai disaster shocked the nation in 1953 and continues to defy belief.

Then aircraft took to our skies and eventually – and perhaps inevitably – were represented among New Zealand's significant disasters. Some occurred in wartime, others when the skies were clear of enemy hazards. Our worst disaster of any kind happened when 257 people were on a carefree excursion to Antarctica and their plane crashed into Mount Erebus.

From the heights of aircraft in flight to the depths of subterranean mining, New Zealand has also experienced several tragic coal-mining and tunnelling disasters. This collection covers the recent Pike River tragedy and also looks back at 1914's Ralph's Mine explosion in Huntly. There are some common features in both events.

Along the way there have been several distinctive, one-off disasters. Mysterious explosions, dramatic flash-floods and tornadoes have caught us off-guard. And that was when we were going about our everyday business.

Leisure activities have also been the setting for tragedy. Yacht races and pleasure cruises have fallen foul of turbulent seas. Mountain climbing jaunts have gone tragically wrong.

In more recent times there have been disasters that are either distinctly Kiwi or related to activities that have become popular on the back of adventure tourism. Cave Creek became a household name when a viewing platform constructed to enable visitors to view New Zealand's pristine native bush environment collapsed.

In a sad irony, 2008's Tongariro canyoning tragedy, when people ventured willingly into what became dangerous waters, echoed the 'New Zealand death' scenario of the pioneering era when so many people drowned because of a lack of roads and bridges.

After the 2011 Christchurch earthquake, we were reminded of the extraordinary courage and unyielding will to carry on displayed by survivors, rescuers and the dispossessed. This book honours those who lost their lives in earthquakes, transport accidents, fires, mining tragedies and other disasters, and recognises the often heroic deeds of rescuers who saved lives and in other ways operated above and beyond the call of duty.

Acknowledgements

The authors would like to thank all those who provided material for this book. In particular, they acknowledge the contributions made by Richard Burton of Tongaporutu; Tony Kokshoorn, Mayor, Grey District; Bernie Monk of Paroa; Cindy Mosey of Nelson; Anna Osborne of Ngahere; Perry Rice, Hamilton City Libraries; and Shirley Slatter, Department of Conservation, Mt Cook.

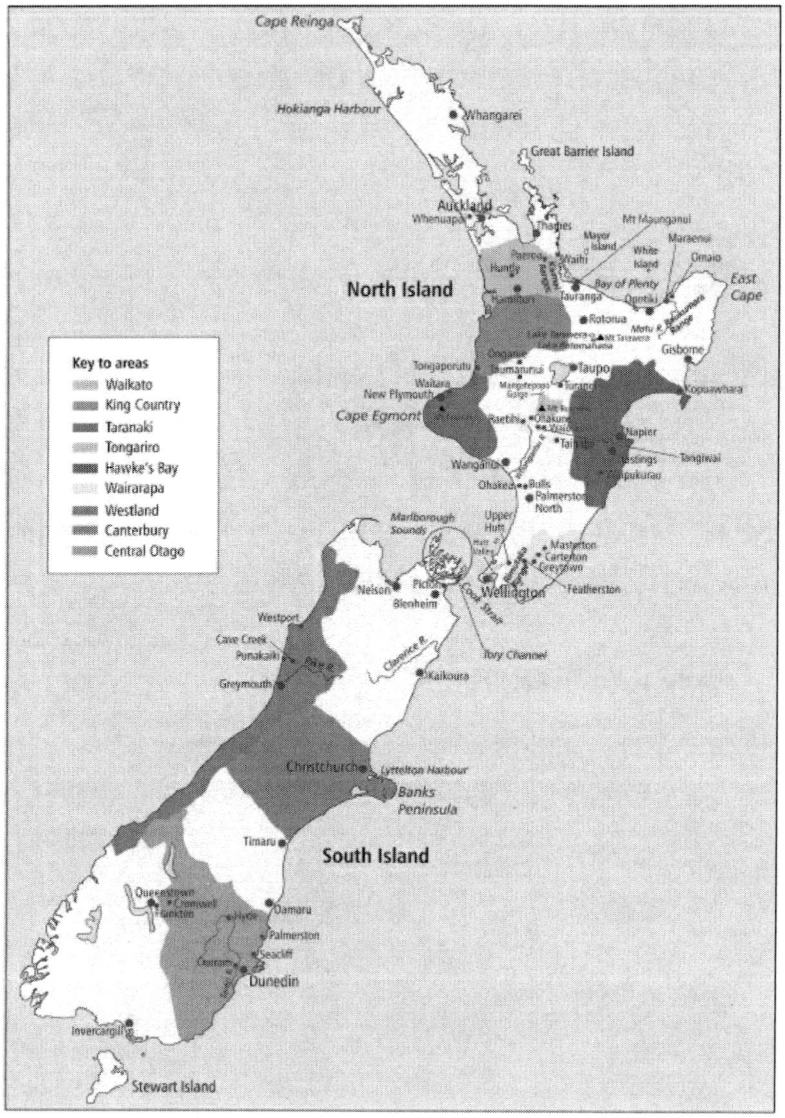
Key to areas
Waikato
King Country
Taranaki
Tongariro
Hawke's Bay
Wairarapa
Westland
Canterbury
Central Otago
Cape Reinga
Hokianga Harbour
Whangarei
Great Barrier Island
Auckland
Whenuapai
Thames
Mt Maunganui
Mayor Island
White Island
Maraenui
Omaio
Waihi
Huntly
Hamilton
Bay of Plenty
Tauranga
Opotiki
East Cape
North Island
Rotorua
Motu R.
Gisborne
Tongaporutu
Taupo
Waitara
New Plymouth
Kopuawhara
Cape Egmont
Napier
Tangiwai
Wanganui
Ohakea
Bulls
Palmerston North
Upper Hutt
Marlborough Sounds
Masterton
Carterton
Greytown
Featherston
Nelson
Picton
Blenheim
Wellington
Cook Strait
Tory Channel
Westport
Cave Creek
Punakaiki
Greymouth
Clarence R.
Kaikoura
Christchurch
Lyttelton Harbour
Banks Peninsula
Timaru
South Island
Queenstown
Cromwell
Oamaru
Palmerston
Seacliff
Dunedin
Invercargill
Stewart Island

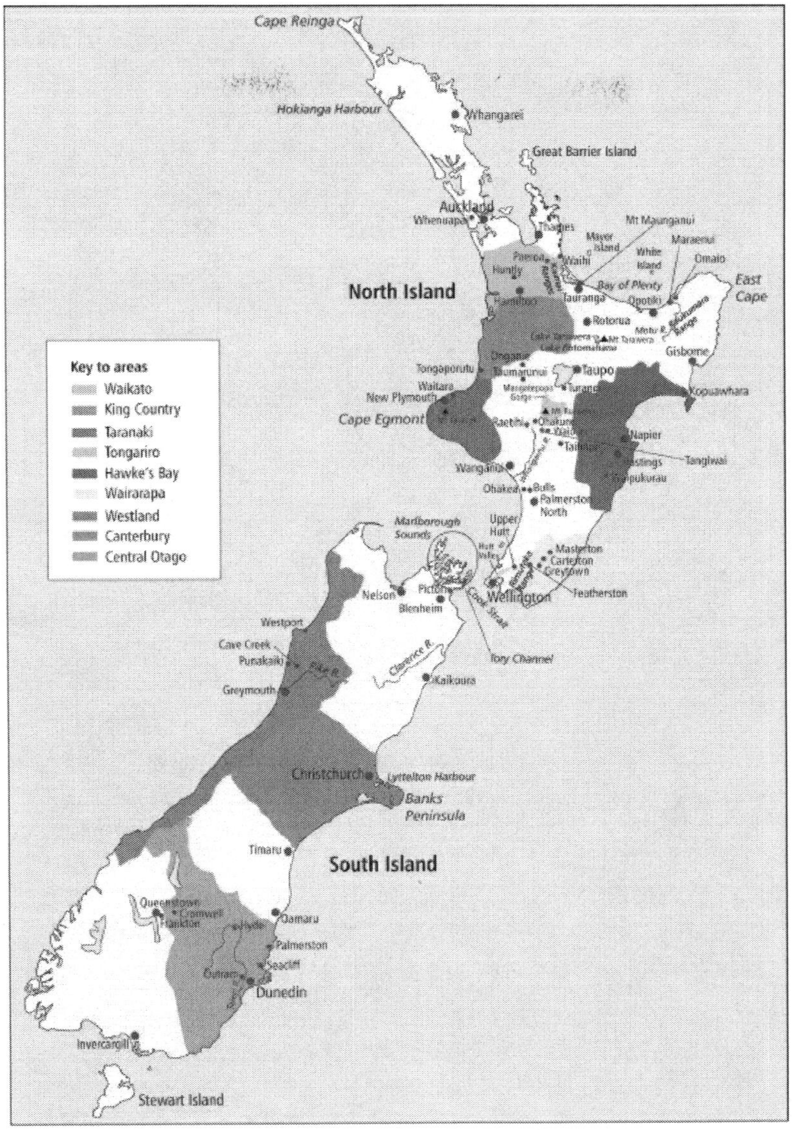
Cape Reinga
Hokianga Harbour
Whangarei
Great Barrier Island
Auckland
Whenuapai
Thames
Mt Maunganui
Mayor Island
Maraenui
White Island
Omaio
Paeroa
Waihi
Huntly
Hamilton
North Island
Bay of Plenty
Tauranga
Opotiki
East Cape
Rotorua
Mt Tarawera
Gisborne
Tongaporutu
Taumarunui
Taupo
Waitara
New Plymouth
Turangi
Kopuawhara
Cape Egmont
Raetihi
Ohakune
Waiouru
Taihape
Napier
Hastings
Tangiwai
Waipukurau
Wanganui
Ohakea
Bulls
Palmerston North
Marlborough Sounds
Upper Hutt
Hutt Valley
Masterton
Carterton
Greytown
Nelson
Picton
Wellington
Featherston
Blenheim
Cook Strait
Tory Channel
Clarence R.
Kaikoura
Westport
Cave Creek
Punakaiki
Greymouth
Christchurch
Lyttelton Harbour
Banks Peninsula
Timaru
South Island
Queenstown
Cromwell
Frankton
Hyde
Oamaru
Palmerston
Seacliff
Outram
Dunedin
Invercargill
Stewart Island
Key to areas
Waikato
King Country
Taranaki
Tongariro
Hawke's Bay
Wairarapa
Westland
Canterbury
Central Otago

1

THE BIG ONE

The Wellington earthquake 1855

In this day and age, earthquakes are very much on our radar. The disastrous Christchurch quake of February 2011 is still fresh in the mind. It registered at 6.3 on the Richter scale and accounted for 185 deaths. It has become part of New Zealand's disaster heritage, our fourth worst in terms of death toll.

Yet there have been many stronger quakes recorded in New Zealand. In 1855 a magnitude 8.2 earthquake hit southern regions of the North Island and the northern parts of the South Island. It was the most powerful quake ever recorded in New Zealand.

'Waiting for the big one' is a phrase commonly used by Wellingtonians in the twenty-first century. They've already had a significant quake in recent times that caused damage but no casualties. Some feel that that represented Wellington's 'turn' on the seismic clock, at least in the meantime. Others are less optimistic though.

In 1848 there was a severe shake in the region, significant enough for many settlers to claim that because it was sharp, it meant that the likelihood of another big tremor was considerably reduced. After the 1848 quake, which saw the destruction of many brick houses and shops, Wellingtonians rebuilt in wood. This movement in favour of wood swept the country. Soon even hotels and churches were fashioned out of wood.

There was certainly plenty of it available.

When steel reinforcing was introduced, brick and concrete came into favour, yet it is considered likely that the low number of brick houses is the reason for New Zealand's comparatively light death toll from quakes, in situations where the strength of earth tremors would be expected to claim more victims.

In the seven years after the 1848 quake, half the settlers in Wellington were new to the town. They obviously had no experience of the 1848 event and when they asked survivors about it they received the general answer that New Zealand seemed to have settled down seismically. They conveniently forgot that Wairarapa, just a short distance to the north, had been assailed by a violent earthquake in 1853 which caused considerable damage and blocked highways. Or perhaps it was the fact that the 1853 quake barely registered in Wellington that led to a growing complacency.

In fact there was a cavalier approach by some Wellingtonians towards earthquakes. The attitude of an Austrian immigrant, Baron Von Alzdorf, a hotelier, was quite common in the burgeoning town. A man with big plans, Baron Von Alzdorf had built a solid two-storeyed hotel of bricks, lath and plaster. He claimed his hotel was earthquake-proof, more so than the many wooden buildings that had gone up after the 1848 quake.

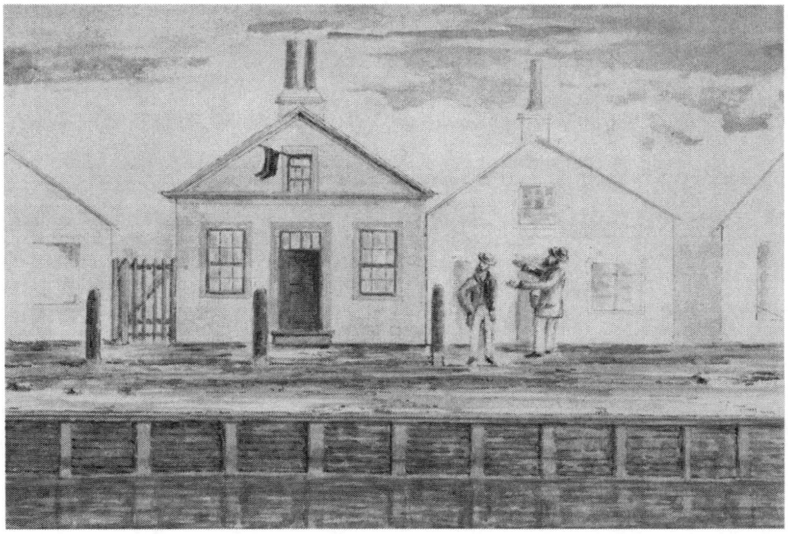

Artist John Pearse's impression of Baron Von Alzdorf's hotel. (Alexander Turnbull Library, Ref: E-455-f-052-2)

Sometime after 9p.m. on the evening of 23 January 1855, the most powerful earthquake ever recorded in this country struck Wellington and the southern regions of the North Island. Even those with a cavalier attitude were startled by the strength of the jolt. The main shock lasted for nearly a minute. More timid Wellingtonians wasted no time in running outside and taking to the streets or other wide open spaces. The more cavalier, like Baron Von Alzdorf, did their best to stand their ground. After the initial jolt the quake returned with a ferocity that sent buildings crashing to earth. After a minute and a half the violent shaking stopped.

As the dust cleared it could be seen that the baron's hotel was a pile of rubble. Sure of the strength of his establishment, he hadn't managed to escape and was dead beneath all that collapsed brick, lath and plaster. It was feared that there would be many more deaths and countless casualties. And yet the only death in Wellington was that of Baron Von Alzdorf, perhaps the one man who felt utterly unassailable should another quake come along. Two people in the Manawatu died when a giant crack opened up in the earth and several Maori (between two and six) were killed when a whare collapsed. To everyone's surprise there were few serious injuries.

Nonetheless, it was a horrifying way to end a weekend of celebrations, commemorating the 15th anniversary of the founding of Wellington. Aftershocks continued to rock the region. They were sufficiently strong to induce many people to stay outdoors, where they remained for the night in tents and on crudely constructed beds. The aftershocks jangled nerves. Someone counted at least 250 in the first eleven hours and they continued for months.

The shock registered at 8.2 on the Richter scale and was felt across virtually all of New Zealand. Centred on Wairarapa, its epicentre was 41.2° S, 175.2° E. Its focal depth was 33 km and maximum intensity MM10. The massive earthquake was highly destructive in Wellington and caused serious damage in Wanganui and Kaikoura. For the duration of the first day an almost continuous vibration was felt by people as far away as New Plymouth when they were sitting or leaning against walls.

The shock registered at 8.2 on the Richter scale and was felt across virtually all of New Zealand.

It seemed odd that such an enormous quake could produce such a small death toll, though it's true that Wellington in 1855 boasted a population of only 6400. Damage to residences and commercial and administrative buildings was considerable. Four-fifths of chimneys were knocked off their pedestals. The grand total of damages amounted to 16,000 pounds which was a lot at the time. The Government offices were completely destroyed, as was the new Union Bank.

The low death toll was certainly a saving grace, but the impact the quake had on land and sea around Wellington and further afield was its major calling card.

The earthquake had originated on the Wairarapa Fault, which was subjected to at least 140 kilometres of movement along the eastern edge of the Rimutaka Range. Close to 5000 square kilometres of land west of the fault was lifted up and tilted. At the southern end of the Rimutaka Range land was uplifted by over six metres. Across Cook Strait the seaward end of the Wairau Valley dropped by over a metre.

Closer to Wellington the ground was raised by 2.7 metres on the western side of Palliser Bay. Uplifting also occurred around Wellington Harbour and the shoreline took on a new perspective. Jetties were now useless because they were so far from the sea. Yet some of the changes were to the town's advantage. A newly exposed stretch of shoreline linking Wellington with the Hutt Valley would provide a shelf to enable railways and roads to join the two conurbations. Additional up-thrust land near Wellington's foreshore provided more opportunities in this and later eras. In fact, much of the central business district was built on land that lay underwater before 1855. And cricket lovers were to be the long-term beneficiaries of an area that used to be part of a waterway that drained into the harbour, but now, thanks to further uplifting, became a sports ground that would eventually be known as the Basin Reserve. The quake also raised the shore platform in Porirua Harbour.

Landslides were another result of the quake. Access between Wellington and Petone was cut off by a massive landslide that blocked the central route to the north and huge landslides slipped off both sides of the Rimutaka Ranges. The Hutt River rose significantly and carried away the principal bridge. At the corner of Willis and Manners streets in Wellington the earth opened up to emit a large amount of slimy mud which covered the main street.

In fact it was responsible for New Zealand's largest-ever locally generated tsunami.

One of the most dramatic results of the 1855 quake was the generation of tsunamis. In fact it was responsible for New Zealand's largest-ever locally generated tsunami. At its highest it rose to 10–11 metres. It affected Cook Strait and Wellington Harbour, where several buildings on the shoreline were flooded. Smaller waves accompanied the many aftershocks. For fully eight hours after the first major shock, the tide rose and receded from the shore every twenty minutes.

The tsunamis were caused by several factors. The land west of the Wairarapa fault line shifted dramatically to the north-east, causing water to inundate the land. Because Wellington Harbour was raised more on the eastern side, the sea moved west, thereby flooding Lambton Quay and other streets. The wave that originated in Cook Strait was probably caused by submarine uplift.

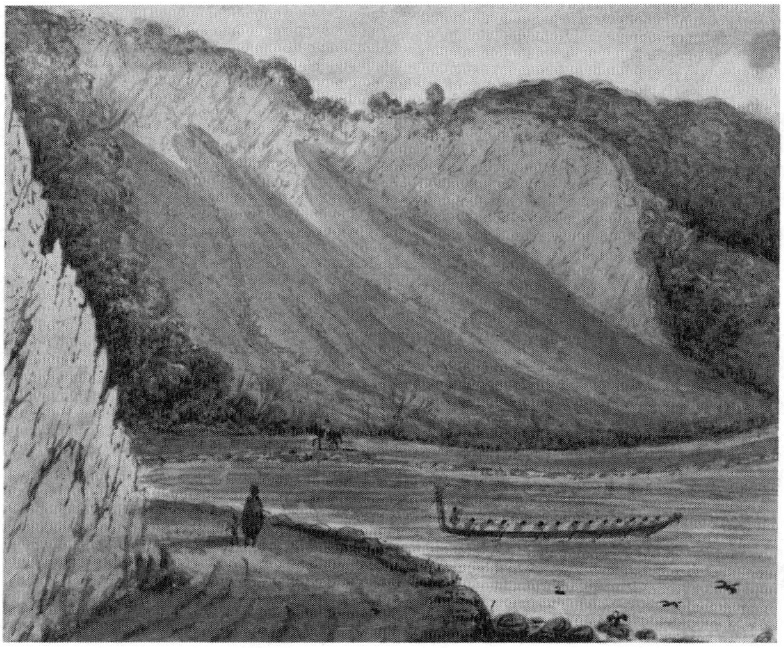

The 1855 earthquake changed the landscape: a depiction by Charles Gold of a large landslide in the Wellington area. (Alexander Turnbull Library, Ref: B-103-016)

One critical factor that prevented Wellington suffering hundreds of casualties in 1855 was the sparse population. Had an 8.2 quake struck Wellington in later decades, the number of deaths would have been considerable as the town grew larger and became a city. Another factor in favour of survival was the time the quake struck. Most adults had yet to retire for the night when, not long after 9p.m., the earth started doing strange things. For this reason children, alerted by their parents, were able to leave their beds and scramble outside before collapsing chimneys and other dangers could cause death or injury. Had the quake struck an hour or two later, who knows what the death and injury toll might have been.

That's not to say that the quake didn't provide horrifying moments for many. A report from a man living in the Hutt Valley described the initial shock, a vertical one, seeming to throw his house in the air. The second one jostled all the chimneys off their foundations and sent them crashing into the rooms. While his two friends who had been visiting were able to clear the building, the man found himself wedged next to a table. His wife returned to assist him but just as the fallen lamp flickered out and total darkness compounded their horror, he saw the chimney tumbling towards him. Luckily a picture frame that fell from the wall landed across his legs just before a good deal of the brickwork from the chimney came down. In this way he avoided serious leg injuries. He and his wife were able to scramble out of the house, to the appalling sound of breaking glass.

There were many reports of such escapes and it was apparent that a good deal of luck rode on the shoulders of Wellingtonians that night. Elsewhere throughout the country the 1855 quake made its mark. In the manner of the 1848 event, it had consequences in regions located as far away as Banks Peninsula in the south and White Island in the north. In Wanganui brick buildings and chimneys were demolished, as they were in Nelson and New Plymouth. In Hawke's Bay and the Bay of Plenty the movement of the earth was severe. It was even noted that a geyser ceased spouting at Taupo.

Smaller settlements were not spared. Paiaka in Horowhenua was badly affected and the people eventually retreated towards the coast and established a new town at Foxton. In the country, farmers in some regions suffered. A sheep farmer at Kekerengu, Marlborough, spoke about members of his family stumbling around like drunken men when the quake struck, forcing them outside into the darkness. They decided to sleep in the woolshed. Later they retreated to a hut on Madcap's Flat and after enduring another night of sharp aftershocks, woke to see their house completely destroyed. The shepherd's house was also levelled.

The lives of such country folk might have been spared, but they were completely disrupted. Without regular provisions they were forced to live off the land. Eels, seagulls and woodhens became part of their diet. A family near Martinborough in the Wairarapa were driven from their destroyed house and ended up living in a calf house.

An initial appraisal of the damage caused in Wellington after the strong 1855 quake made it apparent that there was very much less damage than there had been in 1848. This was attributable to fewer brick houses having been built, and even those with brick exteriors contained wood and iron as bonding agents. Leading locals did their best to play down the severity of the quake anyway. Newspapers limited their coverage and there was little hysterical reportage of the quake. It was considered likely that this tactic was aimed at lessening the panic of the population, given that the 1848 quake had caused an exodus of anxious Wellingtonians.

Some Wellingtonians did leave town while others chose to live under canvas for some time as the aftershocks continued to threaten further damage to their houses. Clearly many were not safe to live in and it was heartening to locals when merchant vessels in the harbour provided shelter for some of the homeless. During this time soldiers of the 65th Regiment offered their services in helping to clear the streets of debris.

Gradually Wellington returned to normal, although it was obvious that certain land movements had stymied some plans for the settlement. The deep-water harbour that was to have been established where the Basin Reserve now stands, and a canal running between Kent and Cambridge terraces to link the harbour with Port Nicholson, were not now possible. Above all, the quake redefined many aspects of the architecture of the town, at least in the short term. Brick and stone lost favour, wood became popular. When Wellington produced 'the largest wooden building in the world' – the Government offices in Lambton Quay – it owed its existence to the fear of earthquakes. Other large wooden buildings went up in Wellington but gradually other materials became popular. It was as if local officials and builders were paying credence to the school of thought that, following the 1855 quake 'the earth would now be at rest for centuries'.

It took only 25 to 30 years for thoughts of building with earthquake-safe materials to die away. Fire resistance became an important consideration in favour of masonry construction. City council regulations in this regard virtually forced the hands of builders. Time passes, memory fades. At the outset of the twentieth century the threat of earthquakes was largely a nonissue. As important an organ as the *New Zealand Official Yearbook* stated quite categorically in the years between 1913 and 1926 that earthquakes in this country were more a matter of scientific interest and less a subject for alarm. Such a stance would prove less than realistic in an earthquake-prone country like New Zealand.

2

OF SHIPWRECKS AND FLOODING

The Great Storm 1868

They called it the Great Storm in 1868. These days they would be more likely to call it the Perfect Storm. Either way, the extreme weather conditions that descended on New Zealand on the third and fourth of February 1868 caused so much death and destruction that it left an indelible impression on the people of the fledgeling colony.

It was probably New Zealand's worst storm, matched or bested only by Cyclone Giselle, the one that helped to sink the inter-island ferry *Wahine.* Ironically, Cyclone Giselle hit New Zealand precisely 100 years after the great storm: 10 April 1968 to be exact. Rather than marvel at the coincidence, however, weather watchers simply accepted the fact as further evidence of our frequently storm-tossed environment. They weren't 100-year events.

In terms of affected areas, the Great Storm of 1868 gnashed its teeth with particular ferocity on the settlement and hinterland of Oamaru. At a time in New Zealand's development when communications and information gathering and sharing were in their infancy, it was recorded that the Great Storm accounted for at least 40 lives. The death toll was likely to have been higher. Who was to say that all was well in remote backwaters and isolated reaches where pioneers lived, cut off from the mainstream?

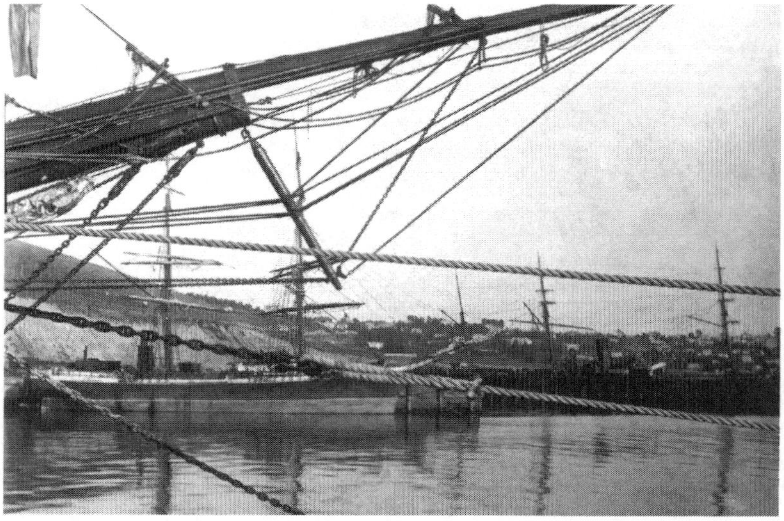

Ships in the port of Oamaru during the latter part of the nineteenth century. (Alexander Turnbull Library, Burton Brothers collection, Box 8, Ref: PAColl-6075-14)

What is known is that on the night of 3 February, the Waiareka Creek, as it ran through Totara Station near Oamaru in a state of ferocious flood, washed away two houses. The Great Storm had played a lethal hand. Intense rainstorms had dumped on North Otago and although locals expected flooding, they were not ready for the flash flood that swept nine souls away.

An entire family of four was wiped out when the first house was hit.

The second house was made of stone and would have been sturdy enough to withstand most floods. Eventually it succumbed to the tumultuous torrent and four residents died. The fifth casualty was thought to be an itinerant passing through who had found a bed for the night.

The port of Oamaru was badly affected by the storm and a ship called *Star of Tasmania* broke adrift in the ungodly seas, ran aground and broke up. Two children, Malcolm and James Baker, were drowned in their berths as the angry waves assailed the ship. Three seamen thought they'd take their chances with the waves and jumped overboard before attempting to swim to shore. All three drowned and while it is known that two of the unfortunate sailors were David Petrie and William Brooks, the name and identity of the third man remained a mystery.

There had been 22 people on board *Star of Tasmania,* including Mrs Baker, wife of a local chemist, her two young sons and a boy named McLean. These passengers were placed in the forecastle which seemed the safest part of the boat, but when the pounding seas smashed the boat's timbers the water rushed in. This was when the young Baker brothers were drowned.

The rest of the contingent of *Star of Tasmania,* a large vessel that had been loading wool for shipment to England, climbed on to the starboard bow where they hung on for dear life. The ship hit the beach stern-first, before swinging around exposing the deck to the lashing waves. As the ship broke up, floating planks of wood presented a hazard to those in the water and Captain Culbert and others suffered injuries.

There had been four ships in the bay at Oamaru when the Great Storm struck. As well as *Star of Tasmania,* another big vessel, *Water Nymph,* was also loading wool bales for export. The other two boats were *Emu* and the ketch *Otago. Water Nymph* withstood the storm surge until early evening, but was eventually driven towards the shore where she came to grief some distance north of *Star of Tasmania.* She slanted towards the beach which enabled all the people on board to scramble to safety.

The third boat to be lost at Oamaru was *Otago,* which had made for the open ocean when the captain had seen the signal hoisted, telling all ships to head for sea. This signal, known as Blue Peter, may have been activated by the harbourmaster as early as 12 noon. *Emu* headed for sea immediately and *Otago* wasn't far behind her. It became a bone of contention that the larger ships, *Star of Tasmania* and *Water Nymph,* didn't respond with similar alacrity, but it was claimed that the seamen on the bigger boats couldn't detect the signal through the increasingly driving rain and murky conditions.

The ketch *Otago* was unlucky. She had travelled five miles out to sea, out of the apparent danger zone when she lost her rudder. The storm drove her back to shore where she foundered near the mouth of Boundary Creek, eight miles north of Oamaru. The boat was completely wrecked but all of the crew were saved.

Dawn uncovered a scene of incredible devastation.

The night passed. Dawn uncovered a scene of incredible devastation. Looking at the shattered ships and debris scattered for miles along the beach, it was regarded as a miracle that only five people had lost their lives. The new Oamaru jetty which had only recently come into operation was now just a pile of twisted iron, attesting to the power of the waves. Seven surf boats were also written off.

The reach of the storm was considerable. There were further drownings to the south of Oamaru. John Chapman, a labourer, lost his life when intense flooding of Whare Creek forced him from an accommodation house and he was swept away. At Tokomairiro just south of Dunedin, Edwin Draper, a butcher, lost his life when he was swept off his horse while trying to save some cattle.

The town of Outram was considered unlikely to survive as a town. Here the flooding of the Taieri was intense but when it started flowing along an old river bed, which now happened to be Outram's main street, the future of the town looked uncertain.

It wasn't just the rural Otago towns that suffered. Dunedin city itself endured serious flooding and Oamaru also had temporary rivers running through its streets – as if the pounding of its port wasn't enough.

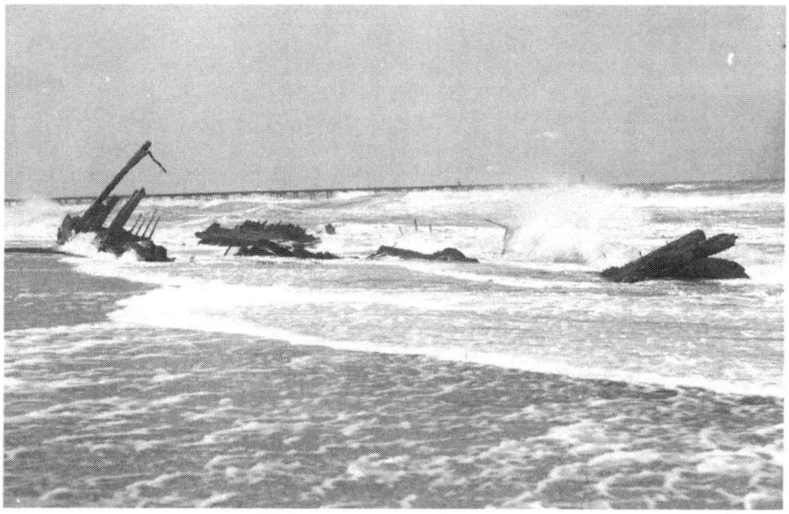

The Great Storm of 1868 left many boats wrecked like this one.
(Alexander Turnbull Library, Ref: 1/1-024448-G)

Five members of a farming family drowned further north at Timaru, and the city of Christchurch was visited by a most unusual flood. Up to early February, Christchurch had received little rainfall. Even when the storm started lashing, Christchurch seemed to escape the worst of the flood – including rainfall. Further north again, the Waimakariri River and the town of Kaiapoi were inundated. The Waimakariri, which used to flow towards Christchurch, broke its banks and sought out its old stamping ground. It linked up with the Avon River at Avonhead and turned what was usually a gentle stream into a raging, yellow-brown torrent which knocked out the Worcester Street bridge and spirited it a long way towards the estuary. Christchurch locals were bowled over, too, by the sheer force of the water and there were some close brushes with drowning. Locals called the lahar-like surge the 'greatest' flood.

During the period of the Great Storm there were 12 shipwrecks. The ship *Echunga* was cast ashore by the storm at Napier and totally wrecked. The crew and nine wharf labourers who happened to be on board were all saved thanks to the bravery of a crew member who swam through the turbulence with a rope and, having secured the line, saw all the others shimmy to shore and safety.

A schooner named *Breeze* foundered at Le Bons Bay, Banks Peninsula, but local residents reacted well and assisted the crew to shore. No lives were lost. This was not the case when a ketch called *Challenge* was washed ashore at Le Bons Bay the following day. It capsized, the mate was drowned and the ketch completely wrecked.

Further north another schooner, *Sea Bird,* was wrecked at Amuri Bluff near Kaikoura. Two more schooners, *Iona* and *Three Sisters,* succumbed to the storm at Lyttelton but fortunately there were no casualties. However, when the steamer *William Miskin* was wrecked at Timaru, one crew member drowned, although there could have been several more fatalities but for a momentary lulling of the waves.

In the North Island the storm lashed Thames and a sudden rise in the levels of the Thames River saw several small boats break their moorings and drift onto the sandspit. The *Glitter,* a cutter, was treated more harshly by the storm, being driven down the gulf and smashing on the beach at Tararu Point. Once again all lives were saved and just when it seemed that Oamaru port would be the only seriously affected mooring in terms of drownings, word came through of more serious loss of life caused by the Great Storm in the far north.

A brig called *Fortune* was hit by the storm ten miles south of the entrance to Hokianga Harbour. The boat was affected by a violent gale that changed direction rapidly. *Fortune* was swept onto rocks and began to break up. Ten crew died at the hands of the Great Storm.

The sole survivor, an able seaman called George Orchard, spoke about being thrown onto the beach in a near unconscious state in weather that featured low, black clouds and a howling gale. When he regained consciousness, Orchard began walking northwards. He had fetched up on the beach in a naked state, the fury of the sea having stripped him of all his clothing. Amongst the brig's wreckage he was able to find sufficient, if unco-ordinated garments, and he now felt more presentable as he forged northwards. He eventually came across a native village where he was granted shelter from the storm, before walking on to Hokianga. He declared that in 25 years of being a mariner he had never encountered a storm such as the one that descended on New Zealand in early February 1868.

The amount of damage caused by the Great Storm was hard for a young country to bear.

The death toll proved to be bad – and the final total could never be known because of New Zealand's scattered and disconnected localities and communities – and the amount of damage caused by the Great Storm was hard for a young country to bear. Roads and bridges were swept away, residential and business properties destroyed. Crops were wiped out and thousands of livestock lost. A contemporary estimation of the cost of the damage ranged between 500,000 and one million pounds.

The Great Storm of 1868 was a typically New Zealand tragedy: climate-based, rain-sodden, befouled by 100-year gales and high seas. Many communities and certainly our ports were totally unprepared for such a tempest. That historians have been able to identify at least 40 deaths is remarkable, given the poor communications and widespread location of a sparse population in 1868.

Many storms are localised. The Great Storm involved most of the country. It was born in the north before sweeping south across the country. It was quite representative. The more you delve into its ferocity, the more significant it proved to be in our history.

In acknowledgement of its importance, Michelanne Forster wrote a play, *The Great Storm of 1868,* which received its first performance at Smiths Grain Store in Oamaru in 2007. Given that Oamaru and its hinterland suffered more than most, it was an appropriate setting. The play was well received and provided an insight into what locals had endured all those years before.

3

NO EASY ESCAPE

The Café Chantant fire 1879

If news were to circulate today that 12 people had died in a café fire in Dunedin, it would produce a reaction of incredulity. In New Zealand's café culture of 2015 such a mishap is beyond comprehension. Had a barista gone bonkers with a flamethrower when someone criticised his long black or flat white? Had the espresso machine short-circuited, or worse, exploded, setting off a conflagration that barred egress from the shop? Had someone forgotten to unlock emergency exits, reneging on their health and safety obligations? Of course there is a considerable disparity between contemporary concepts of café culture and your average New Zealand café of the late 1870s.

The Café Chantant in 1879 Dunedin was a good place for a rollicking night out for those who appreciated that sort of thing. Most didn't. Dunedin, although it had developed into New Zealand's first real city as a result of the discovery of gold, contained many staid and conservative citizens who would have frowned on the rowdy, often bawdy reputation of the Café Chantant.

The café was located in the Octagon in the heart of the city. It occupied the second floor of Ross's Buildings which adjoined the Athenaeum. There were three storeys, with shops on the ground floor and a boarding house and living quarters for the shop owners on the upper floors. People living in Ross's Buildings had mixed feelings about the Café Chantant, which often produced unchecked noise, drunken revelry and murky types loitering in the night.

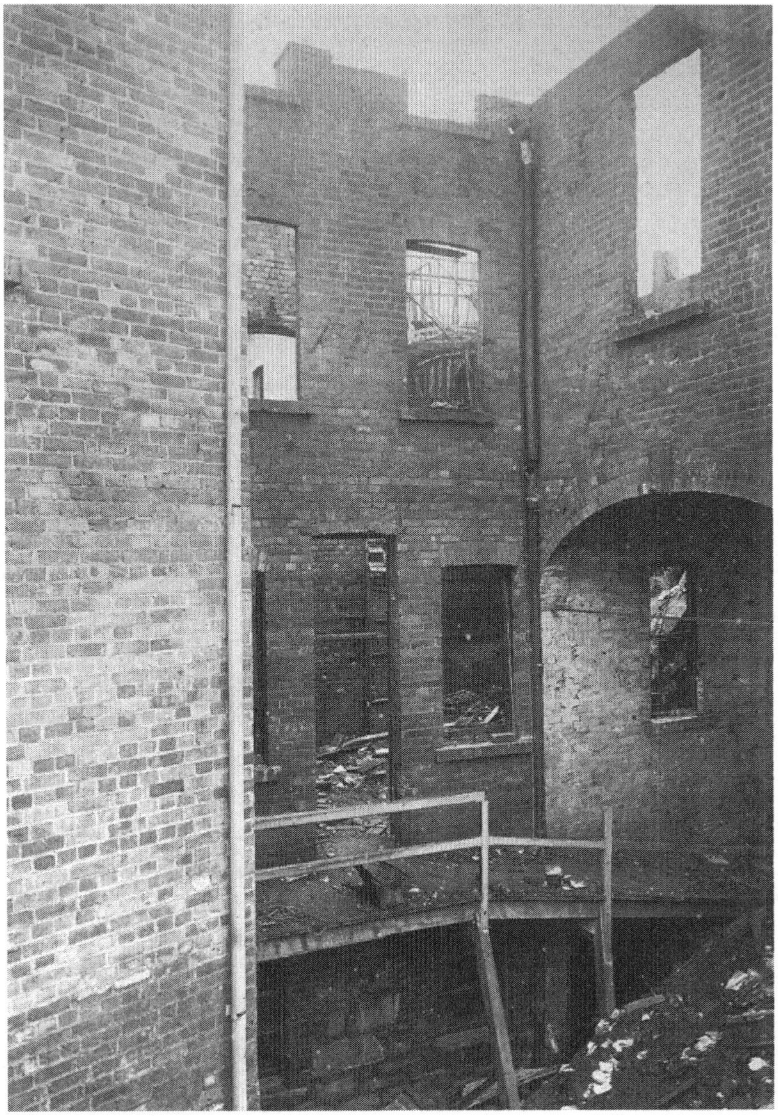

Ross's Buildings in the Octagon were burnt out during the fatal fire. (Hocken Library, University of Otago)

A man named William Waters had arrived in Dunedin from Australia and was responsible for providing stage shows at the café. He also provided plenty of booze and willing company. One of the problems the Dunedin police had with this development was that the café was putting on stage shows every night. And booze and willing company. Complaints of noise and general mayhem reached the ears of police.

Waters was regarded in a poor light by some. He had deserted his first wife in Australia and was now living with another woman in Ross's Buildings. The gold rush, the very reason for Dunedin's exalted position and wealth, also attracted reprobates – opportunists and itinerants – who contrasted vividly with Dunedin's staunch Presbyterian elements. Some of them sailed very close to the wind – and the law.

Café Chantant would not be able to continue in such a debauched and objectionable manner.

Inevitably William Waters received a visit from the police, who announced that the Café Chantant would not be able to continue in such a debauched and objectionable manner. The police were on the verge of taking action against him.

One of the worrying factors about the café was its use of kerosene lanterns for stage lighting. In fact kerosene lanterns were a hazard wherever they were located and in pre-electric days were often the cause of fires. In the Café Chantant, where there was much horsing around and drunken kicking up of heels, it would be easy enough to imagine some high-spirited navvy upending a lantern without even realising it. Alcohol and kerosene were a potentially lethal mix in 1879.

One of William Waters' sidekicks, George Ritchie, the café steward, had the responsibility of filling and maintaining the kerosene lanterns. Ritchie lived in Ross's Buildings and in the early hours of 8 September he heard shouting which roused him from sleep: 'The place is on fire!' It was Waters' voice. Fire bells began ringing, alerting the 50 people who had been sleeping in the building.

The local fire brigade were summoned but from the outset they were found wanting. They lacked the equipment to deal with what had quickly become a large fire. In 1879 the fire-fighting appliance was horse-drawn and while it was found that the horses had been assembled at the fire station, their harness had only been thrown over their backs. It was not secured and was in a bad state of repair.

It was not a good time for a major fire. Two months earlier the fire station had moved its base of operations to a building next to the Town Hall in the Octagon. The transfer from the old fire station had not been completed and essential equipment had not been moved to the new quarters. Precious time was wasted trying to round up the gear. Further frustration occurred when it was found that there were no horses to pull the hook-and-ladder carriages, and the firemen themselves had to provide the motive force.

Many would-be rescuers seemed stunned by the suddenness and speed of the fire. While the fire brigade dithered, the building burned unchecked. Soon occupants began appearing at windows on the upper floors and it became apparent that access to exits was cut off by the flames and smoke. People were soon throwing themselves from third-storey windows, either killing or injuring themselves on the street below. Several died in this manner before someone realised that ladders were available at the nearby Town Hall. Once the ladders were set up, three occupants were rescued before the fire engulfed that part of the building.

The fate of several of the victims was sealed because the seat of the fire was in such a position that many on the second and third floors were cut off from the stairways. The cries of the victims cut through the roar of the fire. Fellow Dunedinites who had come to assist were in a state of panic as the scene became more horrific. After racing around fruitlessly seeking equipment to assist the victims, they simply stood back watching the awful scenes and making sure they were well clear of the building which was now in a state of near-collapse.

There were instances of clear-headedness and heroism, though. Two men were awakened as the fire took hold but were able to scramble out of their smoke-filled room before being asphyxiated. After running to the top of the stairs, they found the passageway burning from end to end. From that point they somehow made it down to the ground floor and safety although neither had any recollection of how they had escaped. Once outside the building, they were informed that several children were still inside. One of the men was able to return and found a young girl whom he carried through the smoke and flames, suffering serious burns himself, before managing to get her clear of the maelstrom. The young man attempted to go back to rescue other children but was driven back by the flames. Three police officers were similarly hindered.

There was the occasional show of ingenuity. One man managed to escape the flames in his room and climbed onto spouting, along which he edged until he came to another room where the window could be opened from the outside. This room was used for drying clothes and the man was able to use a clothes line which he fastened to a bedstead, enabling him to abseil down the wall to the street. The man was able to keep his wits about him, despite the unnerving experience of coming across several suffocated souls sprawled on the passageway floors. Another man in an adjoining room was encouraged to use the same means of escape. Eventually it was reckoned that about ten others found sanctuary by using the clothes line.

One man standing in the street saw a young girl lying prone on a parapet as the flames moved towards her. The man yelled to the girl to jump into the blanket he was holding and after a good deal of encouragement she jumped. Unfortunately she didn't jump out far enough and hit the building which meant she missed the blanket and landed on the pavement.

Her back was injured but she was alive. Another man, J. McGill, had more success when he caught a young woman who jumped from a rear window.

In the morning a scene of devastation greeted onlookers. Nothing was left of Ross's Buildings, just large piles of scattered debris. Twelve people had lost their lives and many were injured. Those of a more judgemental mindset in Dunedin were of the opinion that many may have brought the tragedy on themselves because of their lifestyle. When it was announced that Robert Wilson, the editor of the *Otago Witness,* together with his wife and children, were victims, many Dunedinites bit their tongues. Wilson, his wife – who owned a drapery store in the building – and their six children called Ross's Buildings home.

Robert Wilson was a man of some standing. An Irishman, he had emigrated to the USA where he became well versed in the printing trade. He later worked for several newspapers there before moving to Australia and New Zealand and making his mark. He settled in the large gold-mining town of Inglewood in Victoria and became proprietor of the *Inglewood Advisor,* taking over from no less a personage than Sir Julius Vogel, future premier of New Zealand.

Fire was no friend of Robert Wilson, for when Inglewood's main thoroughfare was all but totally destroyed by fire, Wilson suffered extreme financial hardship. In 1862 he rallied, moved to New Zealand and became the publisher of the venerable *Otago*

Daily Times and, eventually, editor of the *Otago Witness.*

Then came the fire in the Octagon. Robert Wilson, his wife and four of their children perished. The two remaining children, Louisa and Lillie, survived the fire but suffered injuries, burns and trauma.

News of the respectable Wilsons' fate brought a sense of horror to the conservative people of Dunedin. Losing twelve fellow citizens in a single fire was bad enough but when it was realised that half of the victims were from a respectable family, interest in the conflagration increased.

Losing twelve fellow citizens in a sing

Then rumours began circulating regarding William Waters' possible involvement in the fire. It was whispered that he may have deliberately set fire to the building in the interests of collecting an insurance payout. Certainly the local police had already developed doubts about Waters' character, and speculation became rife when it was revealed that the police believed Waters had operated in Australia under another name. The Melbourne *Police Gazette* had published the name of a man, who bore a remarkable likeness to Waters, as a convicted felon. Once again Waters' name arose when locals recalled him negotiating insurance cover with Dunedin business community members, among whom his reputation was tarnished.

Such misgivings were highlighted at the inquest. George Ritchie, the steward of the café, revealed that someone had tampered with the kerosene lanterns and, furthermore, that much of the contents of the kerosene tin had disappeared. Some suggested that Ritchie was trying to shift the blame and focus from himself, as the only person with authority to handle the lanterns and kerosene supplies, to the more shifty Waters.

A jury was assembled to enquire into the twelve fatalities. It reached the conclusion that the fire was the wilful act of William Waters. However, the jury declared that it was not evident that Waters had any intention to cause loss of life. The police then arrested Waters on charges of wilfully setting fire to the building and murdering Robert Wilson. Waters pleaded not guilty.

The subsequent trial by jury in the Supreme Court at Dunedin found Waters not guilty. Lesser charges of arson collapsed too, when no evidence was presented, resulting in a similar verdict. Despite the apparent lack of accountability, the Café Chantant fire remained New Zealand's most devastating fire, in terms of loss of life, until well into the twentieth century.

4

BLOWN OFF THE TRACKS

The Rimutaka rail accident 1880

The Rimutaka Incline was a unique feature of the New Zealand rail system in 1880. It was heralded as a marvellous engineering feat, lauded in some quarters as unique in the world. The climb up the eastern side of the Rimutaka Range, with the line rising 265 metres over a distance of four kilometres, would not have been possible without the use of Fell mountain locomotives, which, as well as conventional wheels, had horizontal inner wheels that gripped the raised centre rail.

The five-kilometre length of railway became world famous. It used the only commercially successful example of the centre rail system, designed by English engineer John Barraclough Fell. The Rimutaka Incline became critical in the running of the main railway between Wairarapa and Wellington. Every passenger service between Wellington and Wairarapa was obliged to straddle the incline.

From the time of its opening in 1878, the incline became an integral part of the New Zealand rail system. It provided an awe-inspiring train ride, although many passengers were pleased when the train reached its less vertiginous destinations on either side of the incline. It had never set out to provide an exciting ride. It was simply a lack of capital that forced engineers to entertain the notion of a steep climb between Cross Creek and Summit station. A more conventional means of getting through and beyond the Rimutakas would have required many tunnels, bridges and massive cuttings. The cost would have been prohibitive.

Many travellers on the Rimutaka Incline railway had misgivings about the safety of the link. At several exposed points along the route, fearsome and sudden wind blasts occasionally assailed the trains as they fought their way up and down the steep slopes. Pessimists were not afraid to express their fears that one day an entire train could be blown off the tracks and plunge into one of the deep valleys between the rugged hills. The loss of life would surely be horrendous.

Many travellers on the Rimutaka Incline railway had misgivings about the safety of the link.

The optimists of course took the contrary view that the sheer weight of the trains, the nuggety Fell engines in particular, would neutralise and absorb any gale Mother Nature might throw at the motive forces and carriages as they edged their way from province to province. There was the reassuring fact that most

Rimutaka Incline trains had four or five Fell engines attached at intervals along the length of the trains. It would take one hell of a wind gust to topple such a train.

Ironically, the four or five Fell engines that were spread along the length of trains were aligned that way to maximise the tractive effect. The fact that this alignment also made trains less vulnerable to the wind was of secondary concern.

On 11 September 1880 a morning train set out from Greytown to Wellington. The small town of Greytown had its own branch line that met the main Wairarapa-Wellington line at Woodside Junction. There were citizens of Greytown who needed to get to Wellington so the train started at the end of a branch line. Soon it linked up with the main line at Woodside, where it picked up more passengers before setting out for the capital.

At the foot of the Rimutaka Incline, at Cross Creek, a Fell engine was added to the train. Two passenger carriages and the baggage car were placed in front of the engine and trailing behind were two wagons of timber and the Fell brake van. It is significant that on this particular day there was only one Fell engine consigned to push the short mixed service up the incline.

Gentlemen were probably reading their daily newspapers, mothers tending to babies and very young children. Several families were off to Wellington for an exciting weekend.

It was a windy day, but then most days in this part of the country experienced some wind. The Fell engine pushed its train willingly and steadily up the grade. All seemed in order. Then the train reached an area on the line known as Siberia. Whether it derived its name from the freezing temperatures normally associated with the Russian wasteland, or the ferocity of the wind, was never established.

Suddenly an unholy north-west gust blew directly across the train's path. The leading carriages were simply blown off the track. It was the sort of rail accident that didn't happen often, if at all. The wooden body of the first carriage was stripped away from its mountings and bogies and the unfortunate passengers were cast like rag dolls against the hillside. Luckily the couplings held, preventing the train being dragged into the yawning valley below.

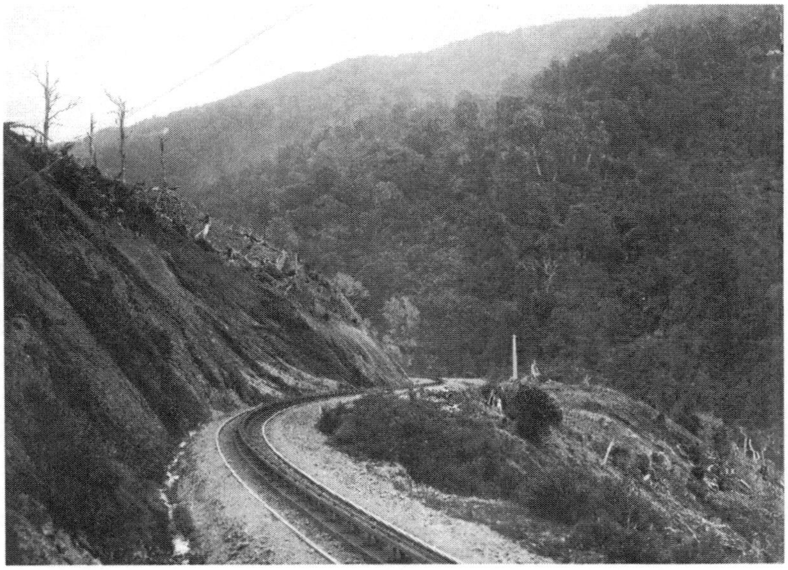

The prominent centre rail on the Rimutaka Incline. It helped keep much of the train on the tracks during the accident. (Alexander Turnbull Library, Ref: 3407 1/2)

At one and the same moment it was possible both to curse the elements and man's desire to push a railway through such an unforgiving landscape, and to bless the solid weight and bearing of the doughty Fell engine – and the vice-like grip of the engine on the raised centre rail. The brake van could also fall back on hardy brakes which gripped the centre rail. In this manner most of the train stayed on the line.

Not only had the rear brake van helped prevent the train from tumbling in its entirety down into the valley, but also, when the rear brakesman uncoupled his van, he was able to run it down the incline to Cross Creek to seek assistance.

It must have been particularly galling for passengers in the second carriage, which dangled suspended over the cliff, destined at any stage to break the link with the rest of the train still on the line. Several men tied ropes to the Fell engine, which were then heaved down towards the second carriage. Passengers grabbed the rope and were pulled to safety this way. The embankment below the line was too precipitous to climb. It was an agonising wait for those passengers who had to bide their time, contemplating a horrendous plunge into the valley if the second carriage broke its coupling or the rope slipped its knot.

It was only when all the passengers had been hauled out of harm's way that the Fell brake van was uncoupled, with the notion of using the van to ease back down the incline to Cross Creek. The van had been supporting what remained of the train but the wind, reminding everyone of its ferocity, lifted the two goods wagons and blew them off the line.

The immediate accident scene was horrifying and gruesome, but not as bad as an artist's impression that was published in the *New Zealand Mail.* The picture showed all the carriages and wagons plunging dramatically into the valley with passengers trailing after them.

The scene was bad enough though. There were many injured passengers and three children had been killed instantly. A fourth, a five-year-old boy, died later from injuries. Some passengers lay stunned on the side of the hill, unconscious for a time. When they roused, the scene that greeted them was like the aftermath of a battle. The dead and wounded lay in all directions, covered in blood. Above them part of the train was suspended in mid-air. Another fearsome gust of wind could, in all probability, send the train crashing onto the injured and into the deep valley.

The survivors crawled to the safety of a nearby cutting where the wind could not reach them. The gale showed little sign of abating. When a rescue train finally made it to the crash site, the rescuers found it necessary to crawl along the track, anchoring themselves to the centre rail. It had been considered prudent to keep the rescue train in a nearby tunnel, for fear that the wind would bowl it, too, off the line. Eventually the rescue party were able to recover three bodies – those of a six-year-old boy, a three-year-old boy and an eleven-year-old girl. Sixteen passengers with injuries ranging from moderate to serious were taken away to hospital.

A young boy was caught by the wind and cast over the embankment.

There were accounts of miraculous escapes – and several heroes. A young boy was caught by the wind and cast over the embankment. Luckily his progress was stayed by passengers in his direct descent path. Had they not caught him he would have tumbled into the valley far below.

Newspaper reports of the accident were initially sensationalist. In lieu of regular and reliable communications, the rumour mill had a field day. An entire passenger train had been blown off the Rimutaka Incline, one report had it. A severe gale had consigned the whole train, which was full of passengers, over a precipice and down to the bottom of the valley, which was recorded as being nearly 100 feet deep.

New Zealand's worst railway disaster of the era created undue excitement in Wellington. Large crowds gathered at the station to witness a special train pulling out to travel to the accident site. It carried medical staff and supplies, breakdown equipment and high-ranking railway officials. Eventually those on the train were able to scotch rumours of massive loss of life, but it was a sobering sight watching the heavily bandaged survivors being carried from the returning special train.

The inquest declared the four deaths to be accidental, with the vagaries of the wind being responsible when the carriages were blown off the line. Two significant outcomes arose from the inquest. Dangerous sections of the line, essentially those exposed to the howling winds, were to have wind shelters built along their length, protecting trains. It was also recommended that when the wind was at its worst, two Fell engines were to be used on the incline. This doubled the chances of trains staying on the line, for the Fell was a weighty beast. The practice of leading trains with vulnerable carriages, where the Fell engine pushed rather than pulled, was frowned upon.

The inquest also heard a passenger accusing the train driver and stoker of drinking brandy before the crash, but there was no foundation to such a scurrilous charge. It was suggested, as a light aside, that most men could understand the driver and stoker partaking of a nerve-settling tot of brandy after the accident, but in truth brandy played no part before or after. And the inquest censured the passenger 'witness' for making up such wild tales that heaped ignominy on the already troubled railways staff.

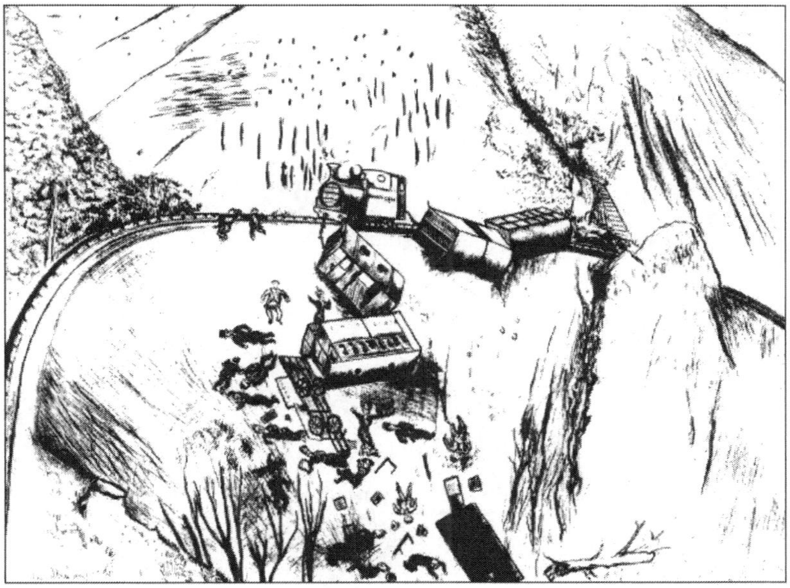

An artist's rather simplistic impression of the Rimutaka crash nevertheless conveys some of its drama. (Sketch reproduced from Evening Post, Alexander Turnbull Library)

After the horror of the 1880 crash, the hope was expressed that this sort of accident would never happen again – at least, not after several long wooden breakwind fences had been constructed to protect trains along wind-prone stretches. No one had told the wind though. In 1888 a severe gale bowled over another mixed train between Pigeon Bush and Featherston. Again only the engine was left standing. The passenger carriages and goods wagons were cast aside. Luckily there was no steep valley on either side of the line and no passengers were killed or injured on this occasion.

Freak gusts of wind continued to be a problem in this part of the North Island. At Makerua on the Manawatu line, a mixed train was blown down a three-metre bank, and although there were some injuries, none was serious.

In October 1936 a railcar travelling south on the main Wairarapa line between Featherston and Pigeon Bush was blown off the tracks by a ferocious blast estimated to be gusting at 128 km per hour. History repeated itself yet again although this time there were no fatalities. Eight passengers were injured. The wind gust struck a short distance from a large wooden breakwind. It was that close.

There were those who considered it fortunate that there were not more accidents on the Rimutaka Incline. When the Rimutaka tunnel was opened in 1955, rendering the incline redundant, many passengers heaved a sigh of relief.

5

THE BIG BANG

The Tarawera eruption 1886

Eleven days before the Tarawera eruption of 1886, passengers travelling from the village of Te Wairoa on a tourist boat across Lake Tarawera with guide Sophia Hinerangi claimed they saw a Maori war canoe. Maori elders considered this to be a waka wairua or spirit canoe. It was an omen of doom to the Maori contingent on the boat, although they recognised it as being merely an apparition. The European travellers thought the canoe was real, although there was something other-worldly about the way it disappeared like a mirage when it was half a mile from the tourist boat.

The Tarawera eruption came as little surprise to some local Maori, particularly after the Maori prophet Tuhoto, speaking after the tourist boat had returned to Te Wairoa, predicted a great disaster with the death of many. Meanwhile tourists continued to visit the area, marvelling at the splendour of the Pink and White Terraces and the scenic beauty of Lake Tarawera and Lake Rotomahana. Tuhoto's predictions faded into the background.

The Pink and White Terraces were regarded as the eighth wonder of the world. Overseas tourists travelled to the area specifically to see the dramatic silicon formations. Those New Zealanders who hadn't seen the terraces often spoke of their desire to do so. Because of the lack of transport networks in New Zealand in 1886, it was obvious that many New Zealanders would never be able to see the glittering staircase and delicate hues of what was possibly the country's leading tourist attraction. For many people the terraces had an almost mythological aura.

Such an impression was only strengthened when, on the night of 10 June 1886, nearby Mount Tarawera exploded in a violent display of volcanic activity. The Pink and White Terraces disappeared as one side of the mountain was blown out. It was believed that the terraces were submerged under vast amounts of volcanic detritus and mud. In the following years there was speculation that the terraces had not been completely destroyed in the massive blast, but because of the ferocious nature of the eruption it would be a difficult task to locate their whereabouts.

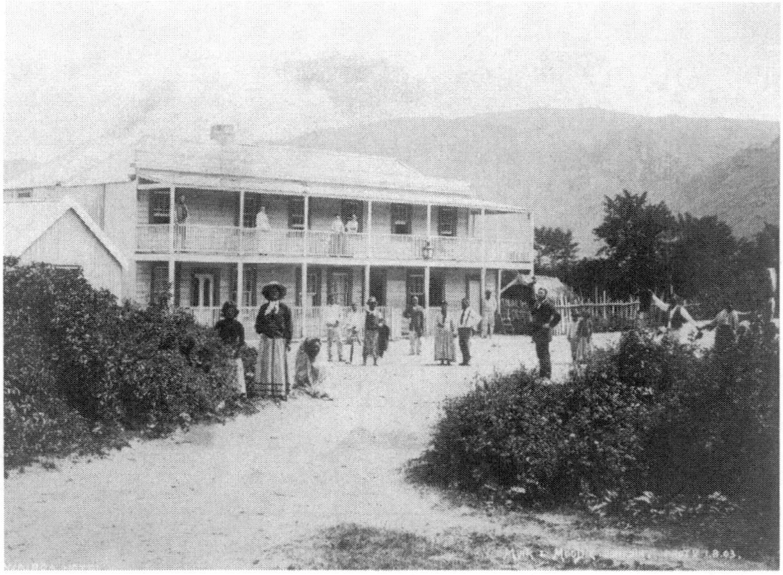

McRae's Hotel, Te Wairoa, before and after the eruption. (Burton Brothers, Alexander Turnbull Library, Ref: 1/2-00333-F; Charles Spencer, Alexander Turnbull Library, Ref:PAColl 7232-3)

The fact that the 1886 Tarawera eruption was strong enough to wipe out the Pink and White Terraces meant that considerable damage was done in the surrounding area. It was an unholy explosion. The blast could be heard for hundreds of miles from the eruption site. Tarawera, a mountain with three craters, was split apart and vast amounts of mud, ash and rocks spewed forth. A series of violent earthquakes followed the initial blast.

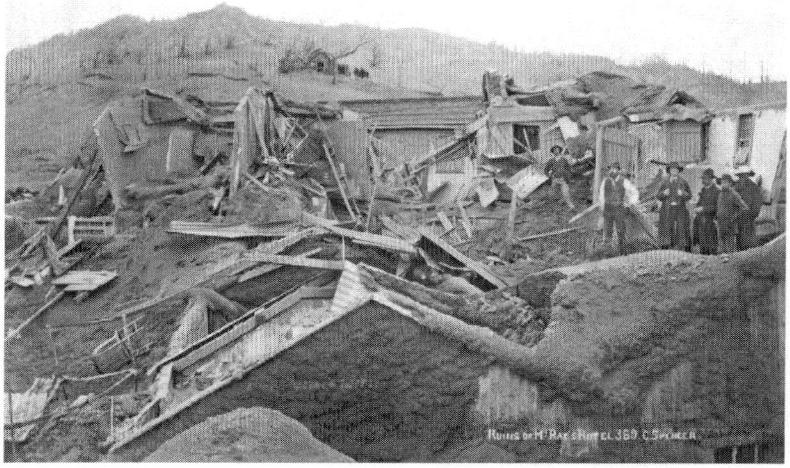

It was such a powerful explosion that it would have caused thousands of human casualties had it occurred in an area of high population density. At the time, the event was compared with that of Mount Vesuvius, which suddenly erupted and destroyed Pompeii. As it was, the Tarawera eruption destroyed seven Maori villages, which disappeared under a rain of rocks, hot ash and mud. The villages of Te Wairoa, Te Ariki and Moura were particularly hard hit and it is considered likely that 147 Maori died. Six Europeans also lost their lives, and the combined death toll of 153 made the Tarawera eruption the most serious disaster of its kind in New Zealand history.

Had the Pink and White Terraces not become such a famous tourist attraction, the toll would have been lower. Local Maori moved to the area when it was realised that they could benefit as tourist guides and boatmen, serving those who had travelled many miles to view the 'eighth wonder of the world'. Then there was the accommodation factor. The government of the day was in the process of surveying a site for a hotel next to the Pink and White Terraces. Had the mountain blown its top a year or two later when the hotel was up and running, the death toll would have soared.

The blast not only claimed many lives – it devastated the surrounding terrain. All plant, animal and bird life was destroyed for miles around. Further afield, the eruption made its presence felt. The booming sound was heard across a vast area, and the earthquakes were felt in far reaches of the North and South Islands. In Auckland locals thought they were hearing artillery fire, and a flash of light in the sky beyond the Manukau Heads was believed to be a distress signal fired by a ship in trouble. Three hundred miles from Tarawera, residents in Nelson, in the north of the South Island, were awakened by loud reports seeming to emanate from vessels miles off the coast. Such sounds were even heard as far south as Christchurch. Many thought that a Russian warship, recently moored in Wellington Harbour, had begun attacking the capital.

A massive, dark cloud was created by the eruption and by the following day it had drifted over the towns of Tauranga and Gisborne. In such places sunlight was temporarily obliterated, turning day into night. Volcanic ash fell in vast quantities over an area calculated to be 6120 square miles. The Bay of Plenty coast was hit hard, and farms in the region had their grass destroyed by thick ash. Many cattle and sheep starved to death.

Closer to the action, the fate of local Tarawera inhabitants was in the lap of the gods. Not only were the Pink and White Terraces obliterated, but a picturesque corner of New Zealand was devastated. The settlement of Te Wairoa hugged the shoreline of Lake Tarawera and had long been regarded as a place of considerable beauty. It functioned largely as a stepping-off point for travellers on their way to visit the terraces and enjoy the bush-fringed lake and towering mountain, long considered dormant. Te Wairoa featured several hotels and guest houses. McRae's Rotomahana Hotel, the Terrace Hotel and Snow's Temperance Hotel provided accommodation for travellers of wet or dry persuasion. There was also a bakehouse, a blacksmith's shop and a flour mill in the commercial area, and a native schoolhouse and teacher's residence, a barman's cottage and an old mission station and church at Te Mu. Several Maori whare (houses) were also located next to the lapping lake waters.

The teacher's residence was occupied by Charles Haszard, the schoolmaster, his wife and son, four daughters and a nephew. Also staying that fateful night were two government surveyors and a Maori woman who was a servant at the mission station.

At about 1a.m. the household was roused by a series of violent earthquakes. Nine miles away, Mount

Tarawera was lighting up the night sky in the throes of eruption. Rather than sense the danger and hurry away from the spectacle, the Haszard household stood on the veranda and marvelled at nature's remarkable pyrotechnics. The moon shone on the lake where the reflection of the fiery glow from the mountain made for a spectacular if unexpected display. Above the mountain itself the sky had turned crimson. This was even more amazing than the Pink and White Terraces.

More ominously, above the crimson glow a dark cloud hovered. Unknown to observers, this was not an ordinary storm cloud but a segment of the mountain that had been uplifted by the ferocity of the blast thousands of feet into the air. Soon earth, mud and rocks were raining down on anything and anyone that lay in its path. At first, survivors considered the fusillade of volcanic stones to be a severe hailstorm. After all, the night had turned bitterly cold.

Miles away, the dramatic light show, now on the wane, had been observed by Captain Stephenson, the skipper of the *Glenelg,* moored in the Bay of Plenty. He described seeing large balls of fire hovering above the land before breaking up into thousands of star-shaped fragments. Back at the eruption site, about an hour after it had begun, total darkness descended. The massive dark cloud had drifted over Te Wairoa, blotting out the mountain's glow and the omnipresent moon. Then the mud started falling.

As the situation worsened, the Haszards and their guests abandoned their shingle-roofed house and took refuge in an adjoining building because its roof and walls were made of iron. It was thought this structure would provide greater protection as the mud, ash and rocks fell and electrical storms continued to strike. Indeed, not long after they had taken shelter in the iron building, a ball of fire struck the chimney of the shingle-roofed main building and in seconds it was blazing from end to end.

Meanwhile the iron roof of the adjoining building had collapsed under the weight of mud and rocks, consigning six of the occupants to an early grave. It was a tragic night for the Haszard family. Charles, the father and schoolmaster, his son Adolphus and daughters Edna and Mona all perished, along with Charles Sutherland Haszard, his nephew.

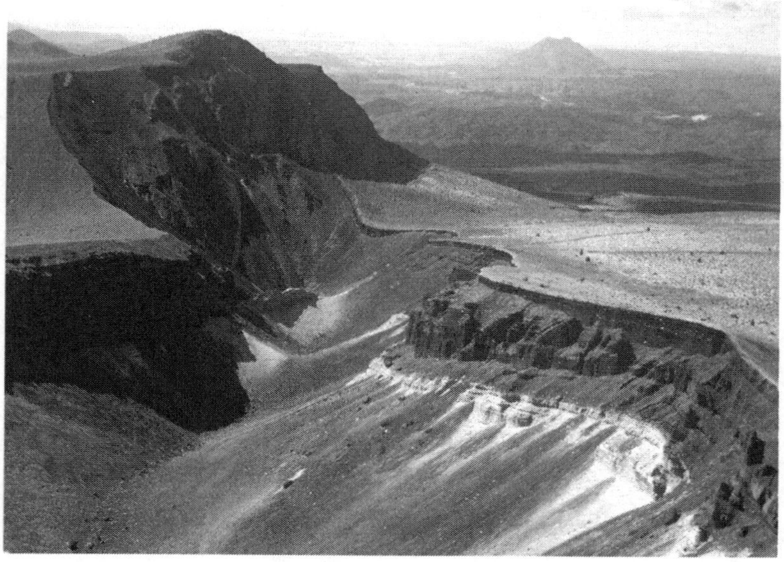

The crater of Mt Tarawera is still a raw, barren gash 130 years after the eruption. (Russell Young)

McRae's Hotel fared a little better. The roof collapsed under the weight of the mud but the downstairs ceiling remained intact until it, too, succumbed to the relentless mud. Most of the occupants were able to escape just before the hotel collapsed completely. Edwin Bainbridge, an English tourist, was unlucky. He ran out of the building just as the balcony subsided and was buried beneath mud and timber.

Several survivors from McRae's found shelter in the strongly built wooden whare belonging to Sophia Hinerangi, a tourist guide. Many locals also sought sanctuary in Sophia's whare, which miraculously remained largely intact as the mud storm played out its course. Had the whare succumbed, the death toll would have been much higher. It was estimated that more than 60 people owed their lives to the sturdy nature of her abode. It is not known how many hens survived in Te Wairoa, but three humans could attribute their survival to the strength of a hen house in which they took refuge.

Once day broke and the hellish night was over, rescue parties from Rotorua and Ohinemutu set out, fearful of what they might find. The villages of Te Tapahoro, Moura, Te Ariki, Totarariki and Waingongongo were completely ruined or buried by mud. Fifteen people died at Te Wairoa, but the rescuers were surprised that so many had survived.

While the loss of life horrified the rescue parties, the rearranged landscape was also a shock to them. They felt as if they had stepped onto another planet. The region was stripped of vegetation. As well as the thick mud and ash that had settled on vast tracts of land, large cracks had opened up. And of course the Pink and White Terraces had disappeared.

Where the terraces used to be, a 100-metre-deep crater had been riven. Within fifteen years the crater filled with water, forming a much larger Lake Rotomahana. Many new geothermal features had appeared, including Waimangu Geyser, the world's largest. Frying Pan Lake, New Zealand's largest hot springs, also emerged after the eruption.

The Tarawera eruption has always held a fascination for New Zealanders, if only for the fact that many details of the devastation were covered up – literally. While accounts of the Haszard family and the plight of others at Te Wairoa have come to light, the obliterating mud, rock and ash consigned many to the fate of almost instant burial. For that reason the final death tallies have always fluctuated.

Some people have mourned the loss of the legendary Pink and White Terraces as deeply as others have mourned the loss of life. There have always been sceptics who, over the years, have refused to believe that everything within cooee of the eruption site was lost forever – and that includes the terraces. Such scepticism has been supported by unusual tales of items remaining intact. A Te Wairoa visitor, having just miraculously rescued Mrs Amelia Haszard, figured a bottle of brandy would revive her spirits. Cautiously the man found his way into one of the ruined hotels where he not only found the bar intact, but not one glass or bottle broken either. Mrs Haszard received her shot of brandy, although it couldn't quell the crushing realisation that her husband and three of her children were dead.

Over the years the disaster site has continued to surrender unsullied objects of life before the 1886 explosion. In 1949 three bottles of wine, intact in every way, were extricated from the pulverised cellar of McRae's Rotomahana Hotel. Some years later a significant part of Te Wairoa village, soon to be known as the Buried Village, was excavated and resurrected. Some of the houses and other structures were brought into the light, one complete with fireplace and a kettle that had remained inert while the explosive seismic and volcanic activity occurred around it.

Finally, the possibility that the Pink and White Terraces were lurking somewhere beneath or beyond the much-changed landscape began to attract the interest of researchers. In 2011 seismic and sonar equipment was assembled in the Waimangu valley to map the floor of Lake Rotomahana. A section of the Pink Terraces (Otukapuarangi) was found, and not long after that amazing discovery, remnants of the White Terraces (Te Tarata) came to light on the lake bed. By 2012 researchers were able to declare that three-quarters of the Pink Terraces were intact, although the fate of the White Terraces was less certain. It was also emphasised that the terraces were located 60 metres below the surface and caked in two metres of mud. Returning them to their status as the 'eighth wonder of the world' would not be easy.

Irrespective of whether the terraces could ever be salvaged as tangible evidence of the worst eruption of its kind in recent New Zealand history, the memories and accounts of that cataclysmic night in 1886 ensure that it will never be forgotten.

6

'THE NEW ZEALAND DEATH'

The Motu River canoe sinking 1900

Even today, the Motu River is regarded as the North Island's last remaining wilderness river. It rises on the slopes of Maungahaumi on the southern side of Raukumara Range, south of Opotiki in the Bay of Plenty. From Maungahaumi the river wends its way through the range and meets the sea near Opotiki on the coast to the north. Much of the Motu watershed is still covered in native forest, and the river itself is unique in that a significant length of its course is confined within a continuous gorge.

It has always been regarded as a lonely backwater, and it wasn't until 1920 that the first modern journey down the river from the Motu Falls to its mouth was achieved by the Fisher brothers and Stan Thorburn.

Part of its charm is its isolation. Even now very few people live on the steep hill country, much still covered in rainforest. Perhaps if proposals in the mid-twentieth century to dam the Motu in the interests of generating hydro-electricity had gone ahead, the area may have been opened up. Hunters have always found plenty of game in the Motu River valley and in more recent times adventure tourism in the form of jet-boating and whitewater rafting have utilised the swiftly flowing waters.

Motu means 'cut off' or 'isolated'. While the definition refers more specifically to the region around the Motu's headwaters where the often impenetrable forest led to it being regarded as the 'middle of nowhere', further down the river isolation was still a factor. Near the confluence of the Motu, a small Maori settlement called Maraenui was big enough in 1900 to have 16 school-age children, but no school. It was isolated.

In getting their children to the nearest school the well-intentioned people of Maraenui were forced to confront the sometimes risky business of having their children cross the Motu River by canoe. One day the canoe flipped over and 18 people drowned.

For 18 souls to die after falling from a capsized canoe in a remote North Island river was a major tragedy. It was a dreadful way to signal the year 1900 in the backwater region dominated by the Motu River.

'The New Zealand death' had struck in its most saddening manner. Sixteen of the 18 victims were children. Death by drowning was so common in earlier eras that the term 'New Zealand death' was coined to categorise it. Because of its bounteous rainfall and broken topography, New Zealand was a nation of many rivers, lakes and floods. And it's an island nation with a long coastline. Even now barely a week passes without reports of drownings, particularly in summer.

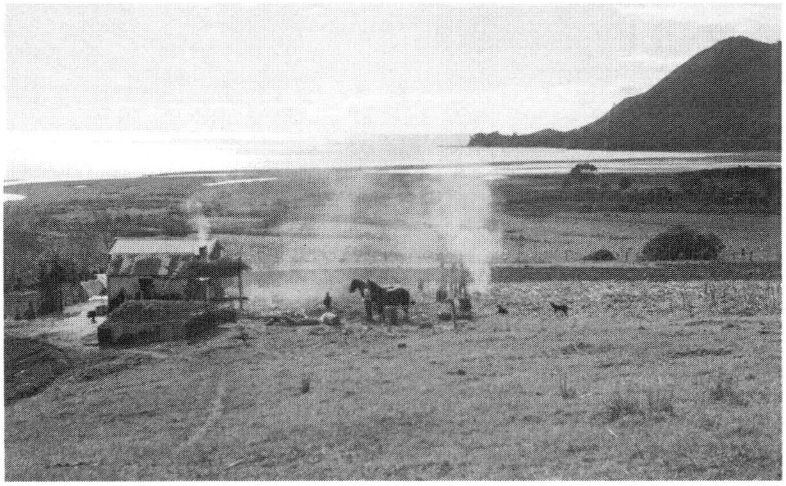

A farmhouse at Maraenui with the Motu River mouth, scene of the tragedy, in the background. (Alexander Turnbull Library, Ref: 1/4-001098-F)

While many contemporary drownings are associated with leisure activities, back in 1900 it was the simple matter of getting from A to B that claimed lives. A lack of roads and bridges often forced New Zealanders to take risks in carrying out their everyday activities. In many parts of the country there were no reliable and safe ferries. People were forced to ford streams and rivers if the water was not too deep. They often did so on horseback. In some situations it was simply a matter of swimming. Many rivers in the Bay of Plenty region could not be forded because of their depth and strong currents.

The tiny settlement of Maraenui is located twenty-odd miles east of Opotiki. Back in 1900 there was no bridge across the Motu River leading to Omaio, another small settlement. This issue became significant when the people of Maraenui wanted their children to attend the public school at Omaio. The school was several miles away, on the other side of the Motu River. To cut down on exhaustive travel time, the children stayed with relatives and friends at Omaio during the school week and returned to Maraenui in the weekends. Their weekends were cut short by the need to get back to Omaio and cross the Motu River on Sundays.

And so it was that on Sunday, 5 August 1900, sixteen children, accompanied by two adults, set out for Omaio. When the Motu River was reached they all climbed into a canoe to make the crossing near the mouth of the river. The river was running high after recent heavy rains so the conditions were challenging.

It wasn't until the next day, when it was noticed that the Maraenui children were not at school, that enquiries were first made. A party from Omaio set out on the Monday morning and found three bodies on the beach. It was thought that they had been washed out to sea from the river mouth and thrown back on to the beach by the surf. It was considered likely that none of the canoe occupants would have survived.

It was a horrible realisation that all the school-age children of Maraenui – those aged between five and 13 – had drowned, along with two adults. Maraenui was traumatised. It was difficult to comprehend the incredible sense of loss. Most families were affected. Some families lost two or more members.

All was speculation as to what happened, although it seemed clear that the woman who drowned lost her life when she plunged into the swollen river in an attempt to save the lives of the children. Her clothes were found on the river bank on the Maraenui side of the Motu, and it was assumed that she hadn't been in the canoe when it foundered.

With the river running high it was considered likely that all the bodies were washed out to sea. Although the river banks were searched, nothing was forthcoming. A tapu was placed on local fishing grounds from Te Kaha on the East Coast to Matata in the Bay of Plenty. The ban was to last for one year and created considerable hardship for Maori living along that stretch of coast, as one of their primary sources of food was unavailable.

The tapu was to last for four years in the more localised area between Tokaputa Point and Whitianga Point and the lower reaches of the Motu River. The prohibition was to be observed and enforced by the Whanau-a-Apanui tribe.

The sea was reluctant to release more bodies. A month after the sinking only six of the 18 victims had been recovered. Many were never found. Coastal currents spirited several souls miles away from the Motu River mouth. Several weeks had passed when the steamer *Terranova* located one of the bodies forty miles from the river mouth. Four more bodies were found closer to home. Paora Arapeta was washed ashore at Tokoroa, near the site of the discovery of Mere Heeni Waewae's body. Mihi Arapeta came ashore at Torere, not far from where another unidentified little girl was discovered. Aporotanga Tuakana, a Maori tohunga, had been called in to help find the bodies. It is said that rainbows appeared, rising from the ocean, and that where the rainbows touched land further bodies were discovered.

A month after the sinking only six of the 18 victims had been recovered.

As bodies were found, a number of elaborate tangi were held at Maraenui. Considerable pressure was placed on the locals, as close to 300 people had to be provided for each day. In a show of support, surrounding settlements donated provisions to help the people of Maraenui through this difficult time. The townsfolk of Opotiki raised money to help pay for provisions as well.

A coroner's inquest relating to the bodies of three of the children was held and the verdict of 'accidentally drowned' was the outcome. Two further bodies were recovered following the inquest. One was that of the man travelling with the children, Pani Retimana, who was found to have been attacked by a shark. A large number of sharks were seen swimming at the mouth of the Motu River at the time of the accident. The canoe itself was found ten miles away at Torere.

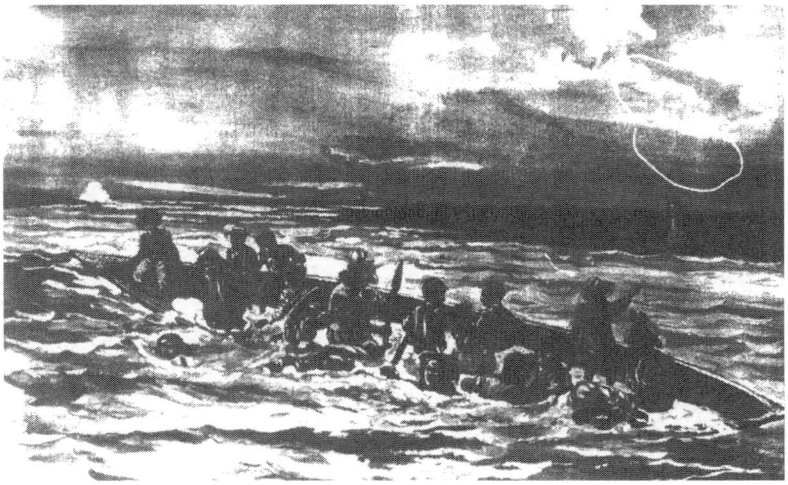

An artist's depiction of the incident near the Motu River mouth. (Sketch reproduced from New Zealand Graphic, Alexander Turnbull Library)

The Motu River canoe disaster was a tragic event. Its impact on the locals was profound and long-lasting. No one witnessed the sinking, apart from the Maori woman who subsequently died herself. There may have been some vague comfort had the sinking been seen by someone who could then report the chain of events to others. But then such a sight would have been both horrific and traumatic. The disaster was protracted, too. The fact that some bodies were never found left a lot of grief unresolved.

Some disasters carry their unhappy memories into history, without certain knowledge and solid evaluation. In the absence of witnesses, those left behind can only speculate and perhaps pray that the demise of those lost was swift and painless. Life lurched on for the people of Maraenui. Time passed – and healed. And then, in 1927, over a quarter of a century after the sinking, Maraenui at last got its own school. There was no need for children to cross the Motu by canoe any more. The bridge across the Motu, linking Maraenui and Omaio, was completed in the same year.

7

THINGS THAT GO BANG IN THE NIGHT

The Upper Hutt explosion 1914

Someone once said that disasters and calamities put small towns on the map. A cynic might see some truth in this claim, although residents of small-town New Zealand would rather their town was remembered for producing locals who climbed the world's highest mountain or split the atom or bred the All Blacks' greatest player.

Upper Hutt, in 1914, was a town. Not so small, but rather a largish town that became a borough that would go on to become a city in 1966. It experienced an event in 1914 that attracted the attention of the rest of New Zealand. Being built close to the flood-prone Hutt River, Upper Hutt would be likely to produce a soul-destroying flood, or so you might imagine. It would have been a serious flood to account for eight deaths though, if that's what it was. The disaster that hit Upper Hutt and put it on the map was more unusual and dramatic than a flood. It was a fire followed by a resounding explosion.

To all intents and purposes it was a regulation store fire. Benge and Pratt's, a grocery/drapery in Main Street caught alight late on Saturday night, 28 March 1914.

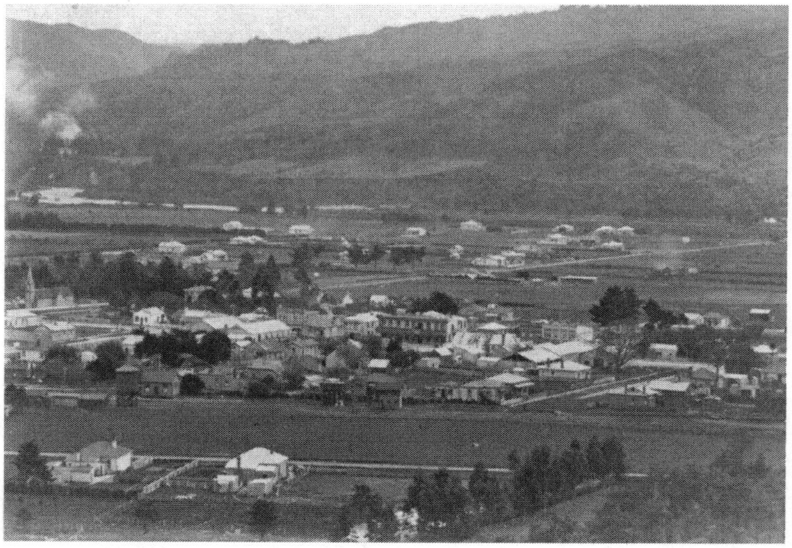

The settlement of Upper Hutt around the time of the explosion in 1914. (Alexander Turnbull Library, Ref: 1/2-110382-F)

It was intense and well involved but there was hope that locals could perhaps quell the blaze. The alarm was initially raised by Mrs Crabtree from the nearby Provincial Hotel. Constable Denis Mahoney, the Upper Hutt policeman, was soon at the scene. Several other townsfolk, always quick to help out when required, raced into the burning building to do what they could. The salvaging of stock was a major objective before the fire hoses could be assembled and played on the blaze. You had to admire the community spirit of those who offered their services in the interests of limiting the effects of the fire. You would eventually curse such selflessness, for without warning a terrible explosion rocked the night and awoke most of Upper Hutt.

The entire premises were wrecked. Four men were killed instantly, another died soon afterwards and there was a sixth death when another Good Samaritan died shortly after being rushed to Wellington Hospital.

Amidst the chaos and carnage the severely injured required hospitalisation as soon as possible. As luck would have it, the midnight train from Wellington had pulled into Upper Hutt station not long before the explosion. William Flynn, the guard on the train, had been one of the first to race to the scene of the fire. While he was helping save stock from the burning shop, the explosion occurred and Flynn was killed outright.

The midnight train was rapidly reassembled to function as a special train to get the injured to Wellington Station, and from there by ambulance to the hospital. The train was driven by W. Grey, with J. Skelton, who had recently piloted the midnight train into Upper Hutt, as fireman. Now they were required to run an errand of mercy in the interests of getting the four severely injured men to hospital. The journey took less than 45 minutes, a record over a stretch of track that usually took more than an hour.

The loss of William Flynn was a shock. He was eventually found buried beneath the wreckage of a collapsed veranda. Another railway employee, George

Taylor, a porter at Upper Hutt station, also lost his life. He had been standing on the balcony of the Provincial Hotel overlooking the fire. He was blown backwards at great force into the wall of the veranda, and although he made it to hospital, he died soon after being admitted.

One of the immediate heroes was Constable Denis Mahoney. He continued saving stock until it was brought to his attention that the building was on the verge of collapsing and there were still several men inside. Under his own steam, Constable Mahoney brought out two men named Scott and Vivian and had just entered the store a third time when the explosion occurred. The store was levelled and large chunks of timber landed over a chain away. It was such an horrendous charge that many felt that no one could survive. Constable Mahoney's body was only recognised because he carried handcuffs.

Constable Mahoney's body was only recognised because he carried handcuffs.

The post office clock stopped at nine minutes past midnight, the exact time of the explosion. Such was its force that it jarred the hands of time into an unmoving state. The postmaster at Upper Hutt, James Comesky, was another early hero who lost his life. He had rushed to the scene in the interests of saving stock and equipment and ended up cast into the street with a heavy window sash and part of a wall on top of him. Rescuers were able to release him and carry him to the billiard saloon, a temporary hospital. After the administration of first aid he was transferred to the special train, but he died before it left the station.

Michael Toohey, like George Taylor, had been standing on the balcony of the Provincial Hotel, where he was a permanent boarder. He had been using a garden hose to spray the roof of the burning building when the explosion blew him backwards with great force. Though grievously injured, he made it to hospital but died early the next morning.

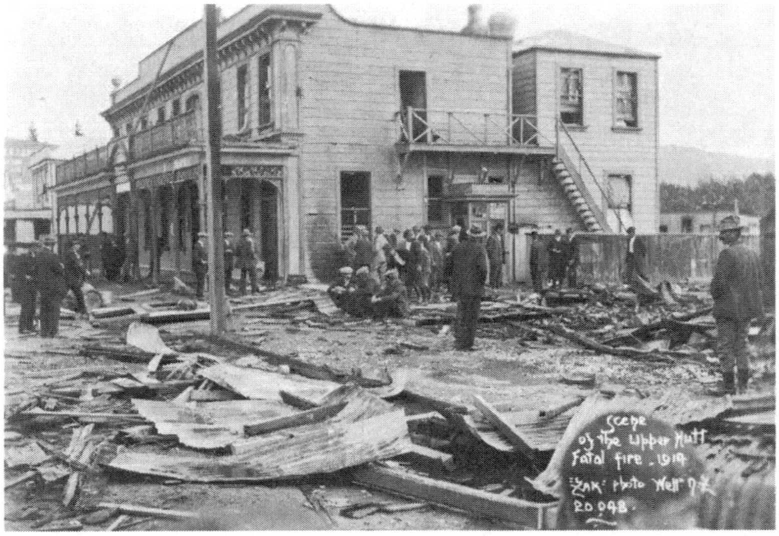

The site of Benge and Pratt's store was a scene of wholesale destruction. The Provincial Hotel next door remained largely unscathed. (Alexander Turnbull Library, Ref: 1/2-022397-F)

The sixth person to die either instantly or in the hours after the explosion was John Vivian, a storeman at Benge and Pratt's. He was near the shop door when the blast occurred, and although he didn't appear to be badly impaired he died before the special train even left the station. Two men, Everard Pelling, a blacksmith's assistant, and Virgil McGovern, a dentist and member of the Upper Hutt Town Board, died later in hospital. Pelling never regained consciousness and died three days after the explosion. McGovern lingered on for nearly a month before succumbing.

Several others were seriously injured by flying debris and were confined to hospital. Others were less affected and had their injuries treated by the doctors summoned from Lower Hutt and elsewhere before returning to their homes. Many townsfolk had miraculous escapes, none more so than J. Hazelwood, storekeeper, who was in his drapery shop affixing sheets of corrugated iron to the back windows in an attempt to thwart the flames from Benge and Pratt's. It was a futile gesture for the shop was completely destroyed. When the blast hit, Hazelwood was caught up in a tangle of twisted iron and burning timber but somehow emerged intact.

Another lucky man was a railway clerk with the surname Broad. He had been helping clear stock from the shop and when he found the heat unbearable, left the building. At that precise moment the explosion occurred. Somehow Broad was not injured. You would not have expected the same outcome for another helper named Thomas who was hurled right across the street, yet he was unharmed. There were others in the vicinity of the store who had similar remarkable escapes.

When you consider that the explosion was heard at Kaiwarra, twenty miles away, and that reports came in of the ground shaking at Lower Hutt and Petone, it was obviously a blast of considerable power. Windows were shattered over a large area – up to half a mile away in places – and many more citizens could have been injured.

The fire itself carried on, largely untrammelled, to burn what was left of Benge and Pratt's before gutting the drapery next door. In what appeared to be a token gesture, the fire was finally quelled early the next morning by a party of fire-fighters with a single hose.

Then the questions started. What had caused the fire, but more significantly, what had led to the explosion? A government analyst, Dr MacLaurin, inspected the ruins. He was to be one of the most important witnesses at the inquest. Detective Sergeant Rawle made enquiries on behalf of the police force. At the outset the shop owners declared there were no explosives on the premises, although the shop was lit by acetylene gas. The gas generator, located in an outside shed, was stated to have been in good running order. The cause of the explosion remained uncertain at this stage.

While such formal investigations carried on, the people of Upper Hutt tried to get back to normal. Sympathy was expressed for those townsfolk who had suffered bereavements or been injured. The ministrations of many of the womenfolk of Upper Hutt were lauded. Some of them had experience in first aid which was put to good use on the night of the disaster and in the weeks that followed.

Then there was the sad business of the funerals. James Comesky, Constable Denis Mahoney, William Flynn and Michael Toohey were interred at St Joseph's Catholic Church in Upper Hutt. It was a joint service and it appeared that the entire town attended. A contingent of uniformed police led the thousand-strong procession. There were 38 constables and nine sergeants. Twenty-four railwaymen in uniform followed, along with the Lower Hutt branch of the Hibernian Society, of which William Flynn had been a member. A number of postal officials also marched.

The other men who died were interred variously at Taita, Wallaceville and Trentham. Virgil McGovern, the last to die, was interred at St Joseph's Cemetery.

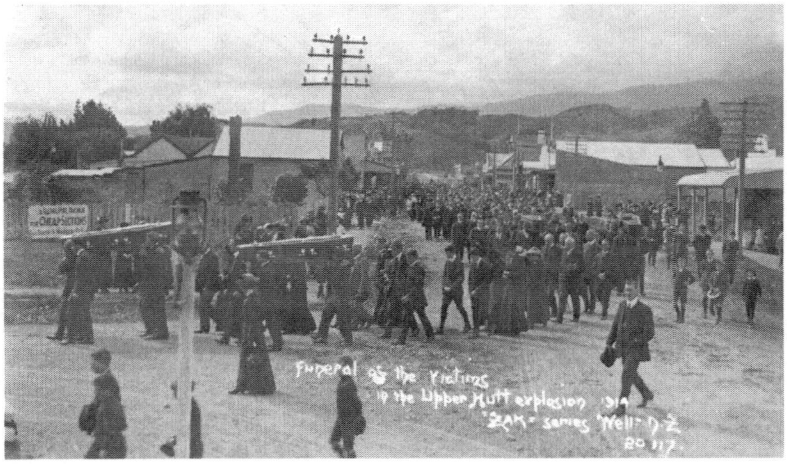

The sombre funeral procession for victims of the 1914 explosion at Benge and Pratt's store. (Alexander Turnbull Library, Ref: 1/2-022396-F)

The inquest into the disaster by the District Coroner was always going to be of significance, for mystery had surrounded both the fire and the explosion. After much deliberation the cause of the fire remained a mystery, although it was revealed that its impact was always going to be profound. Benge and Pratt's was an old wooden building and once it was alight it was considered by the townsfolk to be a lost cause. There wasn't much water available to fight the blaze and such intense fires in those days were rarely bested. In 1914 Upper Hutt had just had a water supply service set up, but lacked a co-ordinated fire brigade. Only one fire hose was available.

The cause of the fire might have been of little moment at the inquest, but what set off the explosion became a vexatious issue. Initially the acetylene gas used to work the lighting in the shop was considered as a cause. Then it was recalled that no one who was in the burning shop before the explosion remarked on the smell of gas. It was also considered unlikely that the nature of the fire would have compromised the gas pipes in the shop. It was not a violent, raging inferno, the type of fire you would expect to be necessary to compromise the gas pipes. These postulations were then declared irrelevant when it was considered that the amount of acetylene required to produce such a massive explosion could not possibly come from the modest in-house gas supplies.

So all eyes turned to the gelignite that Benge and Pratt's had been accustomed to storing upstairs. It was established that 50 lb of gelignite had been received in the shop on 6 February, several weeks before the explosion. Sixteen pounds of the explosive could be accounted for by sales documents, but the rest was not accounted for. No one in the Upper Hutt area came forward to say they had purchased or acquired the balance of the gelignite when enquiries were made after the explosion.

This meant there was a significant amount of gelignite in the shop. Benge and Pratt themselves were not aware of the stockpile in any such quantities, but then they wouldn't have known. Benge didn't take part in the sale of the gelignite and Pratt was not a salesman. He merely ordered goods when required.

At one stage the coroner took note of an utterance made by Albert Cooper, a fifteen-year-old lad who had worked at Benge and Pratt's. He said he knew of the presence of explosives in the shop and mentioned it to others. The police had in their possession a report of Cooper's words to some women before the explosion. Cooper spoke of a 'fine scatter when the powder goes off'. In response, one of the women asked if powder was stored at the shop. Cooper, according to the reports, replied that there was a barrel of the stuff.

The inquest came to the conclusion that the explosion was caused by the gelignite. Thirty-odd pounds had still been on the premises. Only ten pounds would have been enough to produce the sort of explosion that shook Upper Hutt to its foundations.

The Upper Hutt explosion was an unusual disaster. It was the only time in New Zealand's history that significant loss of life had been caused by explosive materials. Despite a rather cavalier approach to the handling and storage of dynamite, gelignite and other dangerous substances displayed by some Kiwis, generally we are cautious around the stuff.

The Upper Hutt explosion gave New Zealanders a glimpse of the destructive force of explosives, shells and ammunition that would become a regular part of the Great War that would soon follow.

8

A PALL OF GLOOM

Ralph's Mine disaster 1914

At 7.20a.m. on 12 September 1914 the ominous sound of an explosion in Ralph's Mine on Raynor Road woke those Huntly residents who weren't already awake. The explosion was so loud that people living in outlying reaches of the district were also jolted from their beds. At the pithead of the mine a massive cloud of black smoke and mine dust hovered over the shaft. For the citizens of the mining community of Huntly, the explosion sounded as bad as it turned out to be. It would end up as the second most serious mine disaster in New Zealand's history. Only the Brunner mining disaster on the West Coast claimed more lives – 65, way back in 1896.

It was initially feared that the Ralph's Mine tally would rival that of the Brunner disaster. Sixty-two men had ventured down the mine only twenty minutes earlier to retrieve rails from a disused section of the mine known as Little Dip. Smoke billowed from the shaft in the centre of town, to be followed by licks of flame that burst high above the pithead. The licks of flame were the most unsettling sight to those who had quickly gathered to wait and were now jammed into the area around the pithead.

There were fears that there would be no survivors, given the severity of the blast. Later it was found that many of the miners had been killed instantly, and the prospect of rescue for those who might have survived was dealt a blow when it was discovered that most of the cages used to transport the miners to and from the surface had been damaged in the blast.

It was only fifteen minutes or so after the explosion that surviving miners were being brought to the surface.

A pall of gloom hung over the would-be rescuers, until a single cage in the main shaft was found still to be functional. Although it seemed like hours, it was only fifteen minutes or so after the explosion that surviving miners were being brought to the surface. Most were severely injured, some having been flung by the blast into solid objects, others badly burned by the flames. Some were affected by both and emerged in a very sorry state, with broken bones and badly burnt flesh hanging in strips from their faces. At least they were alive, although records show that one man later died in hospital.

Escape from the doomed mine had been made doubly difficult by the darkness and the fact that the survivors were not prepared to risk relighting their lamps because of the likely presence of gas still swirling around. One man, adhering to the tenets of what he'd learned in such dire situations, took advantage of the fact that 'good' air in a mine was concentrated near the ground, fell to his hands and knees and crawled out unharmed.

It soon became evident what had probably caused the blast. Ralph's Mine was generally considered safe in those areas where gas didn't seep from the coal deposits and miners wore a naked-flame carbide lamp attached to their cloth caps. In any case, there was a policy that the miner in charge, the only one for whom it was declared appropriate to carry a safety lamp, should lead the way and check the shafts for gas build-ups. On that fateful Saturday, the miner in charge was for some reason at the rear. Perhaps some of that old Kiwi complacency had crept in. After all, Ralph's Mine had been operational since the 1870s, and maybe the workers had come to believe that if they hadn't had a significant explosion by now, they were not likely to.

Miners were stoical chaps. Always had been. It was that very stoicism that got them down the mine in the first place. It was very much a man's world. And now that World War I had broken out, bravery was expected on all fronts.

So what had happened here? The lead man, who should have been wearing the safety lamp, had walked into a dense pocket of firedamp in a disused part of the mine. Firedamp is made up mainly of methane gas, a volatile substance that has accounted for many mining catastrophes in the past. Ralph's Mine's methane was no more friendly than methane anywhere else. When the lead miner attempted to relight his naked-flame lamp after it had unexpectedly gone out, the firedamp ignited. A fireball, fuelled by a cloud of coal dust, raced through the confined shaft towards the pithead.

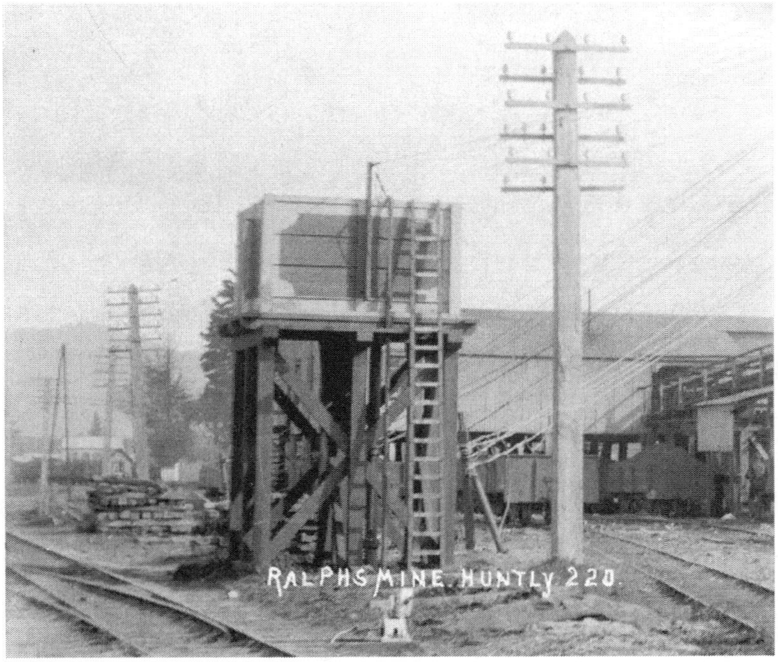

Business as usual. Ralph's Mine, Huntly, in operation several years before the accident. (Alexander Turnbull Library, Ref: 1/2-001763-G)

Some didn't stand a chance; others were able to use the lone surviving shaft cage to escape to the surface. Another group made their way to safety by scrambling through the tangle of tunnels to the nearby Taupiri West mine and clambered up through a ventilation shaft, opened as an airway for Ralph's Mine. This particular escape route was worth its weight in gold, as a significant number of survivors made their escape this way.

At the main shaft the first rescue party was ready as early as 7.45, less than half an hour after the shocking, disorienting roar that woke the town so early on a Saturday morning. Despite their good intentions and obvious bravery, thick smoke and stifling fumes thwarted the first party. A second party was similarly stymied and it became apparent that the mine was on fire. Until the fire was extinguished and the ventilation system repaired, the chances of an effective rescue attempt were unrealistic. Sometimes there's a fine line between bravery and stupidity.

That didn't stop levels of impatience rising in the rescue parties, who were only too aware that their mining comrades were trapped down there, seemingly at arm's length. It was at about this time, while they were still trying to repair the wrecked ventilation system in Huntly, that they realised the ventilation intake to the west might be a possible escape route. Eventually it became evident that the centre of the blast was located roughly halfway between the ventilation intake shaft and the main mine shaft. In the end, eleven miners made their way out of the western ventilation shaft to safety. Most were virtually uninjured after being tossed and tumbled along the tunnel by the force of air.

Rescuers were encouraged by these developments and clambered gingerly down the western shaft. Afterdamp, the gas left following an explosion, thwarted them though, and when they re-entered the shaft they carried canaries in cages to ascertain poison levels in the mine. A pall of gloom descended again.

Canaries were used to detect the presence of deadly carbon monoxide. They reacted to the presence of gas more quickly than humans, and when the birds showed signs of distress miners exited the area speedily.

Back at the entrance to the mine, the crowd that had gathered when the explosion first occurred continued to wait and hope. It was now 5p.m. and the vigil by miners' wives, family members and friends had gone on all day. At this stage the cage reached the surface and a miner, blackened by coal dust, climbed out. He was disoriented but otherwise unhurt. His appearance after nine hours waiting to be rescued raised the hopes of those desperate for news. If someone could emerge unscathed after all that time underground, there might be other unharmed miners waiting to reach the surface. Eventually those waiting dispersed and returned to their homes. It was only then that rescuers brought the bodies of seven badly burned and injured miners to the surface.

Overnight a fresh rescue team combed the mine for survivors – or bodies. As morning broke, four more bodies were brought to the surface. It was long, arduous work but gradually more bodies were recovered, once the fires had been put out and ventilation systems repaired. More searchers were able to enter the main shaft and they found that four of five horses used to pull coal wagons had been killed. The fifth horse made its own way back towards the main shaft and waited patiently until rescuers guided it into the cage and carried it to freedom.

All day Sunday and on through Monday the search continued

The search continued. If a horse could make it out under its own steam then how much better were the chances of humans? All day Sunday and on through Monday the search continued. Nineteen bodies were found, but thirteen had not been accounted for. Tuesday saw the discovery of four more victims.

Fires were still burning in parts of the mine, hampering rescuers, but on Thursday the fires were finally extinguished and larger groups of men were able to join the search. Nevertheless, it was two weeks following the blast before all but one body had been discovered and recovered. A fall of coal had concealed the final body and it wasn't until 27 September that the unfortunate victim was found.

The rescue operation had been a long-winded and dangerous exercise and it was considered fortunate that members of the rescue teams didn't end up on the list of victims. The final death toll of 43 included two men who later died of their injuries. There were only 18 survivors.

The town and district of Huntly was devastated by the disaster. There were 100 children who were made orphans by the accident. Small-town solidarity sprang into action though, and a relief fund was set up for the widows of lost miners.

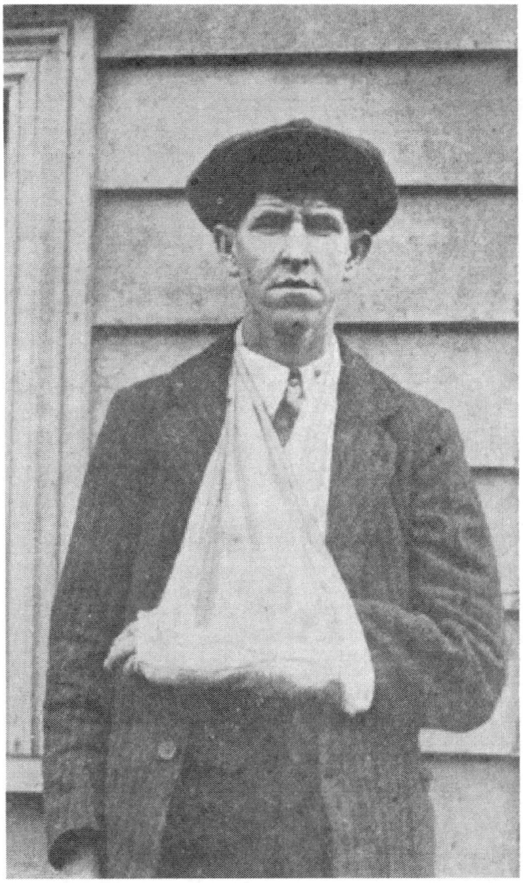

B. Healey, a survivor of the explosion. He was lucky to emerge with only a bruised arm. (Alexander Turnbull Library, Ref: 1/2-028529-F)

Ralph's Mine took some time to return to being a functional unit. Labour disputes delayed the recommencement of work. The mine owners, after it had been established that a naked-flame light had caused the explosion, were ordered to provide safety lamps to the miners. The miners, despite seeing the damage that a naked light could do, objected to using safety lamps because they gave out less light, thus reducing the amount of coal that could be seen. As a consequence, output dropped, and because the miners were on a fixed rate and were only paid for the amount of coal they produced, hard times and lower earnings became urgent issues. In order to compensate, the miners demanded new, more generous rates. An impasse developed.

It seems inconceivable today in the age of OSH and other safety agencies that coal miners habitually wore naked-flame cap lamps to see in the dark. It took the horrible deaths of 43 coal miners to bring about the cry for mandatory use of safety lamps for all miners. The god-awful blast was believed to have been caused by a single miner's naked flame coming into contact with a build-up of firedamp, which consisted mainly of methane gas.

The initial coroner's inquest was found to be one-sided. The miners were not well represented and some felt that important information was held back. The 'ignition of a quantity of gas in number 5 section, causing an explosion of coal dust' was about as far as the initial inquest went.

A later Royal Commission delivered a more democratic process and unearthed many features in the safety aspect of the mine. Probably the main recommendation was that safety lamps should be mandatory for all miners. In fact, a ministerial edict stipulated that naked lights should not be used again. It was rather revealing that safety lamps were previously only used by mine officials and miners in charge. A privileged hierarchy was seen to be in operation.

Further disturbing revelations cast negative aspersions on mining officials. The inspecting engineer of mines told of reports made in December the previous year revealing the presence of gas in Huntly mines. The inspector wrote to the Under-Secretary of Mines in very strong language suggesting that a potentially dangerous situation existed. When several miners suffered burns caused by the ignition of gas, five subsequent warnings to the department should have been acted on.

There were no winners in the Ralph's Mine disaster of 1914. It wasn't even possible to be able to say that a similar accident wouldn't happen again. 'They didn't die in vain' was a mantra that wouldn't be applied to mining accidents. So in 1939, just after another world war had broken out, eleven men were killed in the Glen Afton mine not far down the road. The cause was another build-up of gas, and while the use of safety lamps prevented a fire, all the victims succumbed to asphyxiation.

The 1914 explosion at Ralph's Mine was an accident waiting to happen. The people of Huntly took years to get over it and yet, as the years passed, a new perspective emerged. There was an element of good fortune in what happened in Huntly on Saturday, 12 September 1914. Forty-three men may have died, but because it was a Saturday, only 60-odd men were down the mine. They were working a 'short shift'. On any other working day, 250 miners would have been down at the coal-face. The death toll could have been far worse.

9

WITHOUT A TRACE

The White Island explosion 1914

White Island, off the coast of Whakatane in the Bay of Plenty, is well known to local Maori. Legend has it that when Maui fished up the North Island he stepped onto the new land – but stepped into a fire. In shaking off the flames he created White Island, as the combustible material fell into the sea.

The first recorded European landing on the island was made in 1826 by the missionary brothers, Henry and William Williams. Steam and smoke rose from the ground, evidence of obvious thermal activity. At about the same time, trading ships began landing on the island, where freshly butchered pigs, purchased from Maori, were dunked in hot springs and converted into pork for export and sale in Sydney.

Years passed. In 1848, HMS *Pandora* pulled into White Island and discovered large deposits of crystallised sulphur on the crater floor. Eventually, when the new world needed sulphur for industrial and agricultural purposes (sulphuric acid and superphosphate fertiliser), White Island's resources would be harnessed. Then one day not long after the 1886 Tarawera eruption, people on the mainland noticed a violent eruption of steam and rocks on the island. Obviously if attempts were ever made to mine the sulphur, the volatility of the White Island environment would need to be taken into consideration. White Island is an active andesine stratovolcano and was built up by volcanic activity over 150,000 years. It is the peak of a much larger underwater mountain. Despite the fact that it is New Zealand's most active cone volcano, sporadic attempts to mine the sulphur were made in the 1880s and 1890s. Finally, a fully realised sulphur mining operation on the island was commissioned in February 1914.

In the following months there were two troubling occurrences at the mine. A fireman named John Williams, an employee of the sulphur mining company, died after suffering serious injuries when a retort exploded. The accident happened only three months after the mining operation began. Not long afterwards another fireman, Donald Pye, went missing on the island. No trace of him was ever found, apart from his boots.

Then – disaster. An eruption on White Island killed ten men. It was one of New Zealand's more bizarre calamities. Was it an accident waiting to happen?

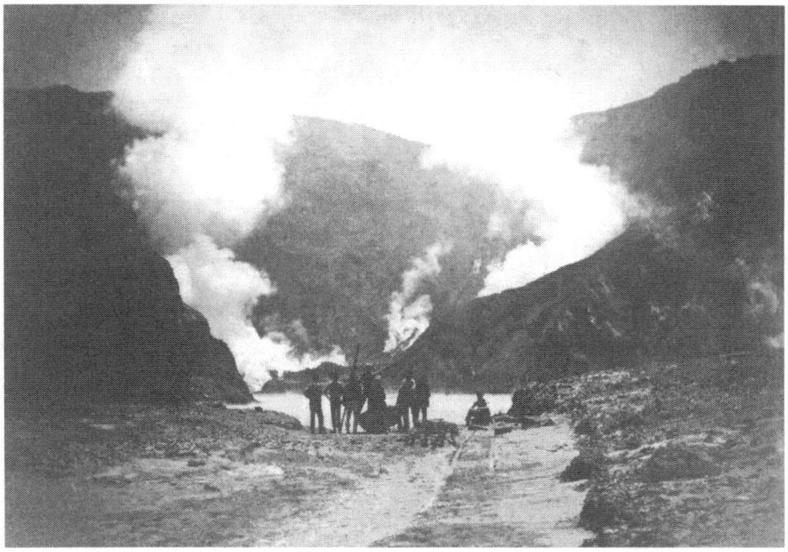

A surreal landscape. Workmen excavating sulphur on White Island before the 1914 explosion. (Alexander Turnbull Library, Ref: 1/4-059933-F)

After the 1914 eruption, the fact that none of the men was ever found and that the true nature of the catastrophe was not uncovered – and will probably never be known – lent a mystique to the event. Originally it was considered likely that an eruption had been the catalyst, but later geologists considered a landslide had been the first of several cataclysmic events. The cliff mass was no longer stable because of the honeycombing effect of steam vents and an earthquake may have set the cliff tumbling. Perhaps the cliff caused a landslide simply because of its inherent weakness.

Eventually the steam burst through and the soft, fallen earth was turned into a mighty wave of boiling mud.

The landslide filled the back of the crater and the water in the crater lake was forced out. Pressure built up after the fallen earth covered the thermal vents. Eventually the steam burst through and the soft, fallen earth was turned into a mighty wave of boiling mud. The lahar or mud flow swept along the crater floor and onto the flat land where the miners' work station and living quarters were located. The lahar had been made more powerful by the masses of rock it collected as it spewed forth. When it encountered buildings and heavy machinery it simply gathered them up and cast them into the sea.

Whether the victims were buried in their beds (the disaster was thought to have occurred at night) and were covered in tonnes of rock and mud, or shunted into the ocean where their bodies were swept away by currents far from the mainland, was never established.

As long as human beings have occupied that part of the North Island that overlooks White Island, it has produced smoke and steam. Even now. On some days the discharge is more pronounced than others. To some that is a good thing. It means that White Island is letting off steam – releasing some of the thermal pressure building up underground. In extreme conditions, such pressure could lead to an eruption on the mainland, or to earthquakes. To others it has always been an unsettling spectacle when the 325-hectare volcanic island sends up steam and smoke clouds. That may not be 'letting off steam', but the precursor of something about to happen on White Island itself.

On 10 September 1914, thick black smoke rising miles into the sky had attracted attention from White Island watchers on the mainland. Sulphur fumes, often detectable from the mainland, were far more pungent than normal. Several other thermal oddities occurred that day; for example, the water in a normally cold spring on a farm near the coast came to the boil. White Island was definitely up to something.

Thoughts turned to the men working at the sulphur quarry. Would they be affected by the worrying signs exhibited by the volcano? To many on the mainland, White Island had always been a god-forsaken place, certainly not an ideal work environment. But it produced bounteous amounts of sulphur and had been regarded as a good investment when the quarry was set up.

A community of sorts had been established on the island. There was a wharf and several surfboats and smaller craft occupied a concrete skidway. If conditions became too unpleasant or unstable on the island, there were means for all workers to put to sea. The camp where the men lived consisted of a works building and a series of wooden bungalows to house the workers. The manager of the quarry lived in his own house, with an accompanying office. There were bunkhouses providing further accommodation, as well as a boiler house, laboratory, retort-house, store and kitchen.

The quarry plant was made up of trucks, rails, reservoir and pipeline, winches, retorts and boilers. So the work site and quarry community were not without their comforts, and once the workers had acclimatised to the strong smell of sulphur and regular earth tremors it was regarded as a bearable work environment. Working on White Island was seen as a good way to save money for there was nothing to spend your money on and trips back to the mainland were infrequent.

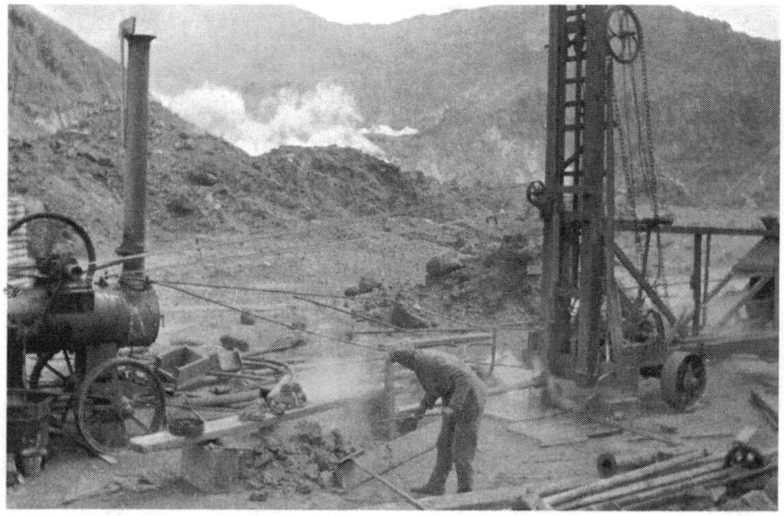

A lone miner working on the island during the 1920s. (Alexander Turnbull Library, Ref: 1/4-059931-F)

In fact, communication with the mainland was rather haphazard. Because of the island's hostile nature and unpleasant smells, not to mention difficulty of access, casual boaties hardly ever visited. Towering cliffs encircled the island and the only gaps in the cliff were at the eastern end of the island. The Northern Steamship Company's pilot, based at Opotiki, was one of the few regular visitors. He carried workers to and from the mainland when shore leave was due. He also visited the island once a week to drop off supplies.

The pilot dropped workers off on the island on 7 September, then visited the periphery of the island again on 15 September. It was late in the day and the weather was foul. The pilot felt a little uneasy that his signal to the camp went unanswered. But then it was likely that the workers were busy on another part of the island and wouldn't detect the signal. It was unusual that some of the men didn't bother to row out to the pilot's boat to pick up the supplies waiting for them.

On his next run to the island on 19 September, the pilot took a dinghy with him. It was his intention to row ashore to see if everything was in order. It didn't take long, once ashore, to realise that things were definitely out of order. A huge section of the cliff had collapsed, creating a new hill in the process, and the camp and wharf had been buried under vast amounts of mud and rock. It was a shocking revelation to the pilot, particularly as there was no sign of life.

It was a shocking revelation to the pilot.

Once the alarm was raised, it was initially thought that all the quarry workers had taken to the boats in an attempt to escape heightened volcanic activity on the island. There was a precedent for this assumption. Several years earlier, sulphur workers had put to sea when the threat of a major eruption was seen to endanger lives. Once the island had settled down, the workers returned to the island and continued mining the sulphur.

However, it soon became apparent to search parties when they landed on the island that this time the situation was far more grave. Part of the volcanic cone had collapsed during an eruption into the island's sulphur lake. Sediment from the cone was converted into massive mud deposits which formed a lahar. The mudflow swept away everything in its path. The workers and their entire community had probably been swept over a headland 50 metres high into the sea.

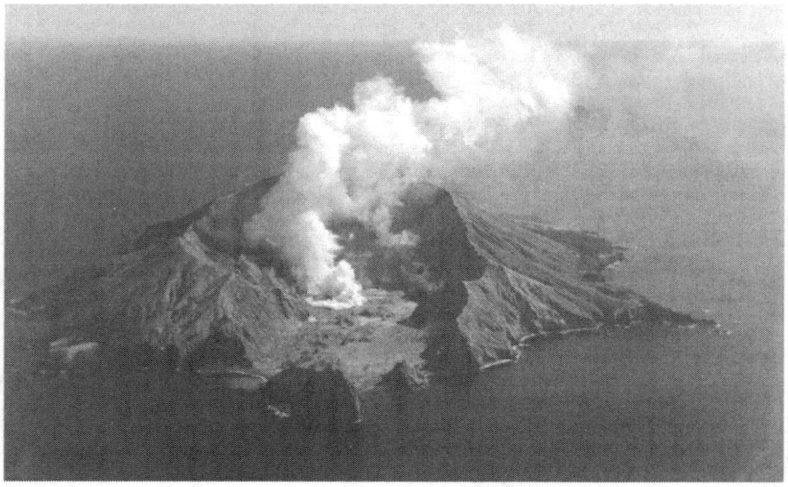

Not to be tampered with: White Island in angry eruption in 1934. (Alexander Turnbull Library 37836 1/2)

Despite a thorough search of the site, no traces of the men were found. Wreckage washed ashore on the mainland and bodies were expected to appear along the Bay of Plenty coast. Back on the island a ray of hope presented itself in the form of the camp cat 'Peter the Great', who was found alive three weeks into the search. Further searches proved fruitless, yet railway sleepers, wharf piles and house timber continued to wash up on mainland beaches. Still no bodies were found.

The victims of the tragedy were listed. Quarry manager A. McKain, S. Young, J. Byrne, W. Donovan, R. Lamb, H. Williams, A. Anderson, R. Waring, L. Kelly and R. Walker disappeared without trace.

The explosion of 1914 brought White Island to national attention. It also intensified the mystery of the place to many New Zealanders. In 1927, when sulphur mining had been reestablished, a series of violent earthquakes hammered the island. This time the workers were able to escape in their boats and remained out on the high seas until the island settled down. Sulphur mining on the island ceased in the early 1930s, by which stage 11,000 tonnes of sulphur had been extracted.

Many wondered if it was worth the effort. Certainly the loss of ten lives in 1914 cast a deep shadow over the White Island sulphur mine.

10

FOR AS FAR AS THE EYE COULD SEE

The Raetihi bushfire 1918

There's a lot to be said for our modern, media-saturated way of life in the twenty-first century. Today the Raetihi fire would receive saturation coverage by a media circus, sending copious updates and breaking news to all points of the compass.

Back in March 1918, World War One was still raging, and the eerie smokescreen that covered much of the lower North Island with its ominous glow of fire set off the wildest imaginings in some New Zealanders' minds. Had the conflict somehow reached New Zealand, and was it now playing out its sinister hand in the back of beyond? Had a new terrible weapon been lobbed onto Raetihi from afar? Or from not so far? Were invasion forces on the march to Wellington, seeking out and destroying all combustible material as they went?

Or perhaps one or more of the central mountains had blown its top, casting ash and smoke miles into the atmosphere, blotting out the sun and causing the molten, fiery regurgitation of mother earth. What was to suggest that the landscape had not been incinerated and blasted by lava?

One woman had somehow come to believe that the volcanic disaster was more widespread than that. Much of Auckland had been levelled. Thousands were dead. Rumour and speculation spread as the strange atmospherics continued to bewilder residents in the capital city. A dense yellow pall hung over Wellington, rendering the hours of late morning dark enough for lights to be kept on. Men who were so inclined were driven to the pubs at opening time, seeking balm to help them cope with the likelihood that the world was in the throes of turning over to die.

In many places it was too dark to work anyway. In Masterton, Featherston and Palmerston North the darkness was even worse than in Wellington. In Carterton factories were closed. It would be too dangerous to try to work in the murk. The pubs in Carterton did a brisk trade as factory workers sought sanctuary and company. If the end of the world was nigh, there was no point worrying about a stiff whisky or two before lunch.

It was sobering though to learn that the smoke hung so thick over the lower North Island that the northbound inter-island ferry from Lyttelton had difficulty negotiating its way through the Wellington Harbour heads.

Eventually the postmaster at Taihape was able to send a message that not only pinpointed the approximate location of the fire, but confirmed that it was in fact a fire and not something as devastating as the rumour-mongers had been concocting. It was devastating enough though. 'Rangataua to Raetihi is a mass of flames and the wires are all down,' he announced. Then all was silent as the message ended abruptly.

Apart from an initial high wind, all was calm at Raetihi on the evening of Monday, 18 March 1918. An hour later the fire first revealed itself over the hills in the direction of Horopito. It developed quickly and by 1a.m. the hills to the rear of the town were ringed by fire. Raetihi had been built in a recess in the middle of dense native bush, and the development of such a fire could be devastating for the town and its population of about 500.

Initially the strong wind was a north-easterly gale, one that would carry the fire safely to the west of Raetihi, but then the vortex changed direction to the north and attacked the town. Dense black smoke made visibility difficult as the townsfolk watched the fire sweep down from the hills and reach the town with great speed.

In no time the northern section of the town had been destroyed. Shops, churches, solicitors' offices, small factories, even the chambers of the Waimarino County Council were wiped out. The ferocity of the fire was such that townsfolk didn't have time to consider firefighting. It wasn't that sort of fire. It was a firestorm. Flight was the only option. Hundreds took refuge in culverts and streams, covering their faces and hands with water or wet cloths.

It was a firestorm. Flight was the only option.

Soon the fire was descending on the back of the town from the eastern ridges and the same ferocious intensity of the fire drove 300 residents into the river under a bridge, where they saw out what was left of a horrific night. The open reaches of the local recreation ground provided sanctuary for others.

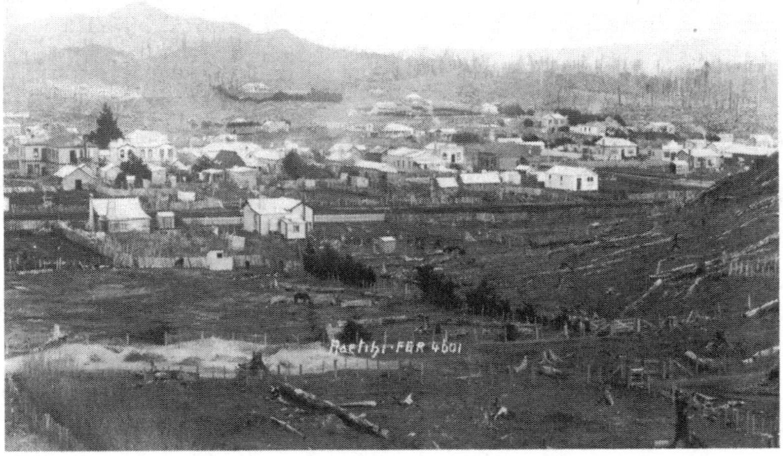

The town of Raetihi showing the effects of the devastating fire.
(Alexander Turnbull Library, Waimarino 5988 1/2)

The fire was heading in the direction of another town, Ohakune, eight miles to the east, but a sudden, merciful wind change and heavy rainfall saved the town from the fate that befell Raetihi.

Amidst the chaos and misfortune, there was one stroke of luck. Not long before the fire, Raetihi had been linked by an eight-mile-long branch railway to the North Island main trunk at Ohakune. At dawn, following a night of hell, Raetihi residents requested a relief train be run down the new branch line. The train arrived in quick time and there were scenes of panic as terrified residents clambered aboard. Some locals had been blinded by the smoke and sparks and had to be dragged onto the relief train. It was reckoned that over 200 Raetihi residents made it out on the first train. The relief train saved many from suffocation. The branch line was a godsend, for the roads beyond Raetihi were impassable.

Railways featured prominently in the conflagration, at a time in New Zealand's history when roads had yet to become the primary means of conveyance. The Minister of Internal Affairs, G. M. Russell, happened to be passing through Ohakune the day after the fire. A deputation of fire survivors met with him and he was able to look into the matter of immediate relief. He also comforted the people by saying that he would contact the Prime Minister, W. F. Massey, from the nearest station. Coincidentally, Massey was himself travelling north by train and when he arrived at Ohakune he spent several hours surveying the situation. While the train was stopped at Ohakune, inspection of the main trunk line to the north was made.

This was prompted by the situation that confronted a goods train when it passed over a culvert. The woodwork that formed part of the culvert's structure was burning and a wagon caught fire as the train was diverted to safety. Meanwhile another express train had been held at Horopito Station all night while the fire raged. The heat caused discomfort but the passengers did their best to ease their plight.

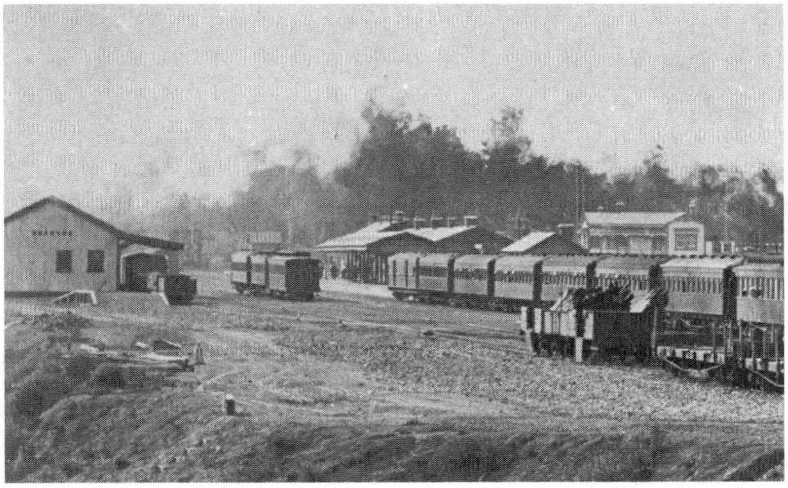

The Auckland to Wellington Express leaving Ohakune Station. A number of key politicians happened to be passing through Ohakune shortly after the fire. (Alexander Turnbull Library, Ref: APG-1516-1/4-G)

The next day a branch-line train carried Raetihi townsfolk from Ohakune back to their town to view the destruction. It was a sobering journey. The town centre appeared to have been ravaged more by the cyclonic winds than by the fire itself. The fire, however, had accounted for the destruction of many shops and private dwellings which were just heaps of tangled ruins. There were some remarkable scenes though. One man had fought hard to save his property, only to see the corner of the building catch fire. At this point he retreated, thinking his fight had been in vain. Now, a day later, he found his house intact, save for the burnt corner.

On the road between Raetihi and Ohakune virtually every building had been levelled. Due to the devastation, it was surmised that many people in the district had lost their lives. The bodies of Mr E. Akerston, a farm manager, his wife and six-month-old daughter were later found in the bush near their burnt-out home. They had only moved to their farm a few weeks earlier. Perhaps their lack of familiarity with the territory contributed to their deaths for, rather than heed the advice of a farm worker and take a short cut to the river, Mr Akerston led his family through an inhospitable stretch. Soon they were completely surrounded by fire and had no chance.

Another farming family survived by climbing into a tank, around which wet blankets were hung. The inside of the tank was padded with wet clothing and for over twelve hours the family endured these gruelling conditions, until merciful rain clouds signalled a heavy downpour and they were able to find their way back to Raetihi.

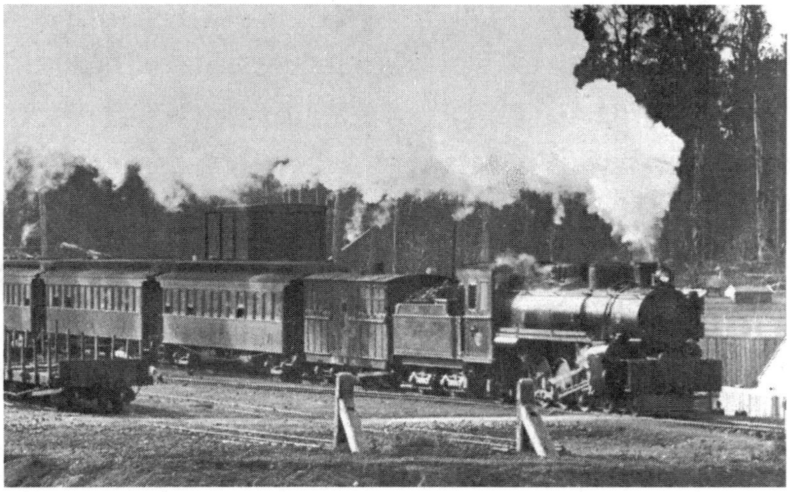

Celebrities were not spared the horrors of the fire. A former All Black, Frank Mitchinson, who was farming at Mangaeturoa, was reported missing. His 600-acre property was blackened by the fire and 500 sheep and two dogs died. Mitchinson made it to the nearby river by wrapping a wet blanket around himself and charging through the encircling fire. Once at the river he climbed onto a floating log and submerged his body in the water as trees burned on both sides of the watercourse.

Some disasters are not measured by death-toll alone. On that score the Raetihi bush fire did not rate highly. It claimed only three fatalities, although many more were injured. The sheer scale of destruction, though, made the Raetihi fire a significant event in New Zealand's young history.

No fewer than eleven sawmills were destroyed.

One hundred residences and many commercial and farming buildings were wiped out. No fewer than eleven sawmills were destroyed, in an area well-known for its timber manufacture. Three hundred locals were left without employment because of the destruction of the mills, and of course there was little or no timber left with which to rebuild their communities. Many locals had to live in tents while the rebuilding process slowly got under way. And the winter of 1918, after the fire, was a harsh, unforgiving one with heavy snowfalls.

The Waimarino district, which included Raetihi, seemed to have been cursed ever since the 1917–18 summer, the hottest in living memory. The bush had been primed to combust. At the same time the area continued to be cleared of bush to make pasture, and the deliberate burning of bush and cleared vegetation meant this was not a fire started by a flicked cigarette, steam locomotive or lightning strikes. All it needed was a wild, dry wind to spread the fires on a broad front.

Following the fire and the horrendous winter, the great influenza epidemic further battered the region. Raetihi and the Waimarino district in general suffered more than other parts of the country, and it was suggested that the inhalation of smoke and ash from the bushfires rendered many locals susceptible to the bug. The harsh winter hadn't helped either. The district took years to recover from the events of 1918.

It took an extreme optimist to see some good in the fact that the Raetihi bushfire had occurred in a relatively remote and lightly populated part of the North Island. In a more densely populated area the death toll could have been much higher.

11

BUT FOR A BOULDER

The Ongarue rail accident 1923

Major disasters often produce tales of miraculous escape. Rail disasters frequently feature instances of passengers swapping seats, sometimes to their detriment. In the Ongarue disaster, members of a Maori rugby team had been booked in a specially reserved carriage near the front of the train.

At Auckland Station they had settled into their seats and were looking forward to a jolly, rousing journey. A few minutes before the train pulled out, an official asked the team to move back to a first-class car near the middle of the train. The reason for this was never revealed, although it was likely such a move would free up seating in the carriage nearer the engine, where at some stations down the line easier egress and boarding could be achieved. Despite protests by the rugby players, they moved back to the other carriage. Such a move saved many of their lives.

Another group who were very fortunate were members of the Scandal Theatrical Company who found their reserved carriage was not at the head of the Auckland to Wellington express when they boarded at Te Awamutu. It was located further back. There were other travellers who were not so fortunate. They lost their lives when the train hit a landslide just south of Ongarue, near Taumarunui.

The crash represented New Zealand's first significant loss of life involving the railway network. There had been mishaps before, but not on this scale. The seriousness of the damage to the express was such that far more fatalities could have been expected. Some of the carriages splintered like matchwood when they ran and telescoped into one another.

Heavy rain was the culprit. It was midwinter in the heart of the King Country and the skies had opened up, making the hills above the main trunk line – always slip-prone – vulnerable. It is not recorded when the massive slip came down but it presented an impenetrable obstacle for the express as it moved down a slight incline not long before dawn. The incline led to a sharp curve in the track. High banks at this point meant the train driver and fireman could not see the terrible obstacle that lay ahead. When the engine's headlight revealed the slip after the train had turned the corner, the driver immediately applied the brakes to their maximum extent.

The train was only ten feet from the landslide when the brakes were applied, so inevitably it hit the slip. It was recorded that the engine may have ploughed its way through largely unscathed, but for the presence of a large boulder in the middle of the slip which came to rest between the rails. The chances of this happening were considered extremely unlucky, and although the engine managed to carry the boulder for some distance on its cowcatcher at the front of the train, the boulder eventually threw the engine, its tender and the following postal van off the line where they came to rest against the bank of the rail cutting.

The boulder eventually threw the engine, its tender and the following postal van off the line.

It was unavoidable that the carriages would telescope. While the engine, tender and postal van avoided this calamity, the second carriage wasn't so lucky. It was driven by the forward momentum of the train through the first carriage with startling force. When it had finished carving its way through the first carriage, there was only half a metre separating the front doors of the first and second carriages. The roof of the first carriage was splintered.

With such immediate devastation, it was inevitable there would be many casualties. The worst cases were in the first carriage. It contained 30 passengers, several of whom were among the 12 who were killed outright. The second carriage had been full and many were injured. The third carriage was more fortunate. Not only was it carrying a mere seven or eight passengers, but it was lifted skyward by the force and came to rest at an angle on top of the second carriage. The remaining carriages missed the terrible concussion created by the carriages closest to the engine, and apart from general dishevelment and broken windows, remained relatively intact.

At the head of the train, the driver and fireman were blasted, burnt and scalded by steam from the broken steam injector. Heavy bruising was also inflicted on the train crew. In the following postal van, the three postal workers were fortunate that their wagon was of a sturdier disposition than the carriages, being more recently built. Apart from a few minor injuries they emerged relatively unscathed.

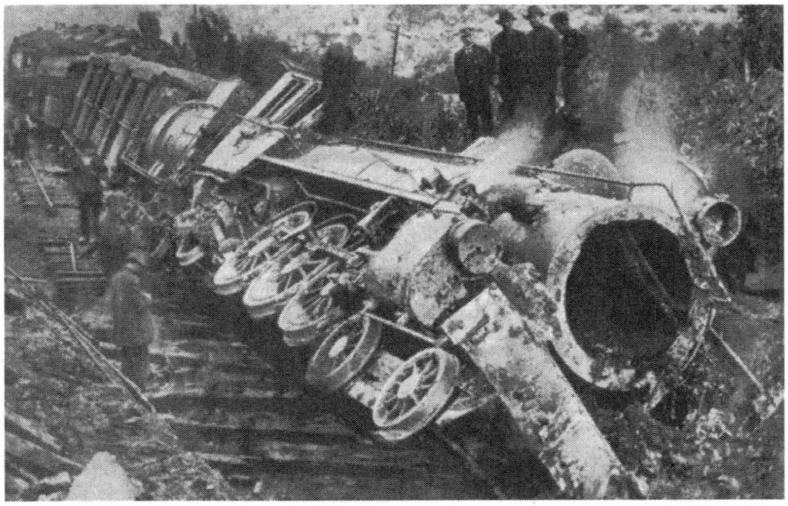

The Auckland-Wellington Express derailed at Ongarue. Seventeen people died. (Graham Stewart)

As if the express was not in a big enough plight, a gas container used to provide carriage lighting burst into flames beneath the number three carriage. The prospect of a fire was a ghastly thought, with many passengers still pinned in their seats. One quick-thinking man leapt down to where the fire had broken out and began heaping soil and stones on the flames. Very soon another slip careered down the hillside. Was there further agony in store? Fortunately it was a small slip. Moreover, it was a friendly one, for it fell in such a way that it smothered the gas and stopped the fire spreading.

Time passed slowly as dawn broke on a desolate scene. Before help arrived, those passengers who were relatively unscathed did their best to rescue trapped passengers. One man in the third carriage had spent nearly half an hour groping around in the darkness, contemplating the damage and debris, listening to the anguished cries of those still trapped and injured. Then, much to his relief, the guard and a relief gang began breaking through the wall of the carriage with hammers, saws and whatever they could utilise as implements. Soon passengers were being lifted to safety.

The alarm had been raised by an uninjured passenger who had run down the line to the nearby settlement of Ongarue. As luck would have it, there was a medical doctor on the train. Dr Bathgate had his work cut out though, with so many injuries to tend to. Luckily his medical bag contained a goodly supply of sedatives and he was able to ease the plight of those victims in extreme pain.

A nearby house belonging to a ganger on the railway was seconded and functioned as a temporary hospital. The injured were tended to by a group of women, including a nurse who had served in the First World War. Many of the injured had suffered head injuries. Eventually these casualties, together with those who had been treated back at the scene of the derailment, were accounted for, and a special train from Taumarunui ferried them to the local railway station. Here residents who owned cars transferred them to Taumarunui Hospital. It was a Herculean humanitarian effort, tempered by the knowledge that three casualties died before reaching hospital.

Seventeen passengers died and 28 were injured.

When the final terrible tallies of those killed or injured were made, the Ongarue tragedy was declared to be New Zealand Railways' first accident that led to major loss of life. Seventeen passengers died and 28 were injured. There had been earlier fatal rail accidents. The Rimutaka Incline accident of 1880 caused the deaths of four children and injured 21 passengers. In 1899 two excursion trains smashed into each other at Rakaia Station and three young women and a child were killed and 11 injured. In 1914 there was a similar accident at Whangamarino station on the North Island main trunk in which three passengers died and five were injured. In an accident that was remarkably similar to the Ongarue incident, a southbound train ploughed into a large landslide just north of Mataroa in 1918. Two postal workers in the wrecked postal van were killed, as were two passengers in the first carriage. Eight passengers suffered serious injuries.

But the Ongarue accident in July 1923 jolted the nation. Because train travel was the dominant means of transport at the time, a certain amount of trepidation was experienced by the man – and woman – in the street. The Mataroa accident had involved the express hitting a landslide too. Was a pattern beginning to form?

The Board of Enquiry into the accident cleared the Railways Department of any possible negligence in causing the tragedy. Massive rainfall had led to the slip, a causative factor over which the department had no control. However, the suggestion was made that carriages on the North Island main trunk be suitably strengthened to reduce the amount of telescoping and crushing of cars, should further such incidents occur.

Muted criticism was directed at the Railways Department for procrastinating over the decision to replace gas lamps with electric lights. It was sheer luck that a serious fire failed to break out under the third carriage, solely due to the small landslide which smothered the fire erupting from the gas containers. If nothing else, the Ongarue tragedy hastened the installation of electric lighting instead of gas.

There was a certain naiveté relating to the Ongarue crash. New Zealand was not used to experiencing such a calamity. And yet an earlier and not dissimilar incident not far south of Ongarue should have set alarm bells ringing.

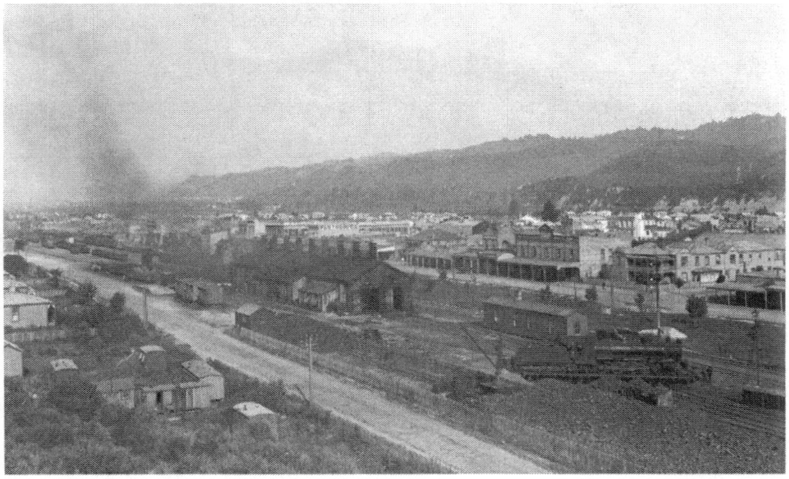

Looking over Taumarunui Station, from where the injured were transferred to the local hospital. (Alexander Turnbull Library, Ref: APG-1114-1/2-G)

Little more than a day before the Ongarue crash, a violent, prolonged rainstorm had swept across the Waikato and King Country. A great wedge of hillside was affected by the deluge and it oozed down onto the line at a tiny sawmilling settlement called Owhango. A goods train hit the landslide and once the locomotive was derailed, the Main Trunk line between Auckland and Wellington was impassable. Owhango and Ongarue were only twenty miles apart. Because the heavy rain at Owhango came from the same weather system that caused the slip at Ongarue, it's not unreasonable to think that the rail authorities might have been more vigilant.

By the time the doomed express set out, the line had been cleared at Owhango, although the blockage had led to departure delays from Auckland. The weather was still bad, but at least the express was travelling at reduced speed as a concession. Some proffered the opinion that perhaps the express should not have been travelling at all. What was to prevent another slip on the line, given the persistent nature of the rainfall?

In those days New Zealanders put their faith in rail authorities. If the latter declared 'safe passage' on the Main Trunk, passengers could rest easy. And on 6 July 1923 they could even get a good night's sleep in the express's sleeping carriages at the back of the train. So much so, that when the train hit the slip and all that destruction and loss of life occurred, some of the sleeper passengers remained blithely unaware of the horrible events unfolding. It was only when they were woken by survivors from the affected part of the train, requesting bed linen to be used as bandages, that the unaffected stirred and, to their credit, ventured forth to assist the injured.

The Ongarue crash, with its 17 deaths, is still the third most serious accident to occur on the New Zealand rail system. Tangiwai with 151 fatalities and the Hyde disaster with 21 are listed ahead of it. And to think that, but for a boulder in the middle of the slip, the disaster might not have happened at all.

12

BAD VIBRATIONS

The Napier earthquake 1931

When the Napier earthquake first struck, at 10.48a.m. on 3 February 1931, the merchant ship *Taranaki* was being loaded with frozen meat in the port. It was already a hot summer's day and the gangs found the conditions so sapping they were taking a break from the manual slog. Suddenly, the whole ship began to vibrate as if the engines were building up pressure. Soon the vibrations became violent and so unsettling that some of the men began to panic. Was the engine room on the verge of blowing up completely?

Then the men looked towards the Napier shoreline. A strange grey dust cloud was seen rising all along the length of the bay. The dust came from collapsing buildings and other city fixtures as the infamous Hawke's Bay earthquake played out its deadly hand. The vibrations on the *Taranaki* were the result of the quake making its presence felt.

In the heart of Napier the quake struck viciously. Two-storey buildings collapsed everywhere. In fact, it was later reckoned that every building standing more than a single storey high was bowled over. As the buildings collapsed, the dust clouds rose. Many residents were trapped in falling buildings. Many didn't make it out. Others were killed by falling masonry and shop façades. There was pandemonium as people rushed around, doing their best to escape the hazards.

Many ran to the nearby beach, away from collapsing buildings. Some structures were totally destroyed. In the nurses' home at Napier Public Hospital, a dozen nurses who had been working the night shift were killed in their beds while sleeping. Schools collapsed entombing schoolchildren and teachers. Workers died as the quake levelled several factories. In an old folks' home, 14 men over the age of 80 lost their lives. Hotels, business premises, shops and private residences were no match for the 7.8 quake. Away from the centre of town, in the lee of the nearby hills, landslides covered houses or killed people as they sought safety in their own backyards.

It was suggested that those residents who were seated in motor cars when the quake struck would be better protected than most. Then reports came in of drivers crushed at the wheel as cars succumbed like tin cans to falling walls and building façades in the downtown area. Even motorists outside the central business area were not spared. Cars driving beneath Napier's Bluff Hill were flattened by falling rock and landslides.

Many died in the quake itself, but then fire broke out in the centre of the city which spread quickly and lethally. Many of those who were still alive, but trapped in the debris, lost their lives to the fire. The quake had severed the water mains and there was no water with which to fight the flames. Napier burned for 36 hours.

Napier burned for 36 hours.

The Napier fire started in chemist shops where gas jets were kept burning to melt the wax used to seal prescriptions. Elsewhere ruptured gas mains provided the spark. With the water mains rendered useless, firemen threw their intake hoses into the sea, but this provided only a token amount of water and the fires burned on.

Rescue attempts were fragmented and it was regarded as something of a godsend that HMS *Veronica* had arrived at Napier port little more than 90 minutes earlier. The captain of the *Veronica,* H. L. Morgan, was on deck when the loud roar and violent shock of the earthquake hit. He could see the wharf twist and buckle, buildings collapse and the roads open up with great fissures. Cars and drivers were swallowed up. Railway lines were thrown into crazy alignments. It was obvious to Captain Morgan that there would be hundreds of casualties.

He and a team of his men walked gingerly into town from the wharf, providing assurance where possible and generally appraising the situation. After several harrowing hours walking the broken streets of Napier, Captain Morgan was able to send out the first coherent report on the situation. In a radio message to the Auckland naval base he declared that virtually all of the stone and brick buildings had been destroyed. Wooden buildings had fared little better and now they were at the mercy of the developing fire. The failure of the water supply was hindering the fire brigade. Captain Morgan and his men organised a food depot, as well as several makeshift hospitals for the hundreds of injured. HMS *Veronica* was set up as an x-ray centre.

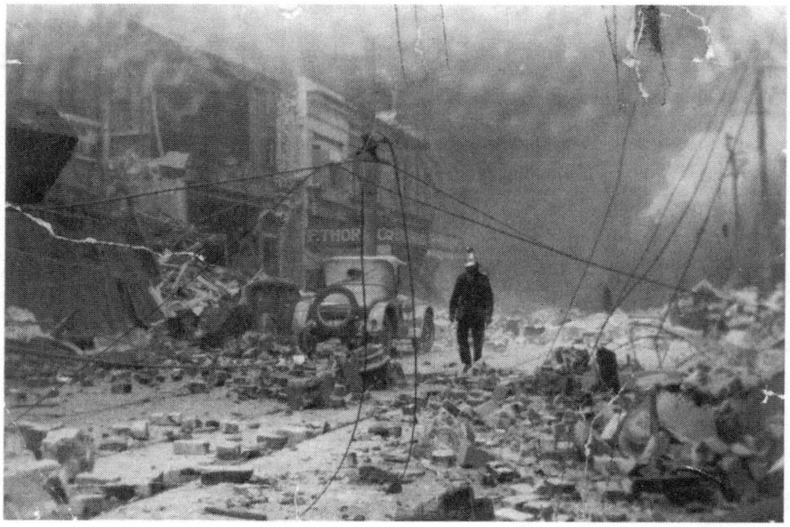

A lone policeman contemplates the horror caused by the Napier earthquake. (Alexander Turnbull Library, Ref: 1/2-139885-F)

Some wound-dressing stations had to be established in the open spaces, given the lack of safe, surviving buildings. Operations were carried out in such situations and such was the need and number of patients, doctors carried on into the night, guided by the lights of acetylene flares and the headlights of those cars that hadn't been crushed or buried. Luckily the rain stayed away, but it was probable that some operations would have continued even if the skies had opened up.

Other areas of Hawke's Bay were badly affected by the quake. Hastings was in ruins too, although fire was not the problem there that it was in Napier. The scenes in the ruined city of Napier reminded some observers of battlefields in World War One. These images would have been enhanced as the two cities were evacuated and navy officers began blowing up buildings that were leaning at crazy angles, destined to collapse and possibly cause more deaths among the rescuers. Dynamite was also used to create a huge hole at the Napier cemetery so that 54 coffins could be buried.

Official statistics tabulating the numbers of dead and injured took some time to materialise. There was often confusion over who had survived, for many were still listed as missing. James Durning, for example, was listed as a victim. He was buried in the rubble for three days and then rescued only to find his name listed in the obituary section of a local newspaper. He went on to live well into his 80s. Three days after the quake, a 90-year-old man was discovered alive beneath the ruins of an old folks' home.

There were other miracles amidst the death and destruction. A chimney collapsed at the Salvation Army maternity home and crashed to earth a few centimetres from five babies in their bassinets. And there were inevitably heroes. The sailors from HMS *Veronica* were among the first, providing much-needed leadership and direction. Firemen, policemen, doctors and nurses worked long and hard to ensure the death toll didn't become even more serious. People forgot their own circumstances – and often safety – to deal with the mounting casualties. A Hastings doctor worked tirelessly in the operating theatre despite learning that his daughter had been an early victim.

Survivors were evacuated from affected areas. Convoys of cars, trucks and buses eased down the damaged highways towards safety. Special trains ran as far as they could on the main east coast line. Many of the injured were spirited out of the area by train. The trains also brought in back-up medical staff from Wellington. Further medical staff were shipped in by naval vessels from Auckland. It was no surprise to most that, on viewing the levels of destruction, many thousands would require medical treatment.

Another problem – one that contributed to the speed of the evacuation – was the damage to sewerage systems and the attendant fear that typhoid would break out. Many citizens became homeless and were obliged to improvise in terms of shelter and a bed for the night. They were at the mercy of the elements and deteriorating hygiene conditions.

On the first night after the quake there were few who considered it safe to sleep indoors, so many survivors slept under the stars. The Army handed out tents, and makeshift shelters utilising sacking sprang up in many backyards. Luckily it was a balmy February evening. Had the night turned to rain, not only would misery have been compounded but collateral sickness would surely have followed.

Hunger was also a problem. Food supplies were often buried in shops and houses. Bakeries and butcheries were difficult to locate in the wasteland, let alone their food supplies. Basic bread was eventually supplied every day by bakeries in those outlying towns less affected, but the obvious solution to the plight of the people was to evacuate as many of them as possible.

Aftershocks continued and many residents felt it best to be away from the threat of further collapsing structures. To confirm their fears, a massive jolt struck as night fell. It was strong enough to throw people over like ninepins. Many buildings that had been partially bowled by the major quake now crumbled completely. Even those buildings that had been considered by some to be salvageable bit the dust.

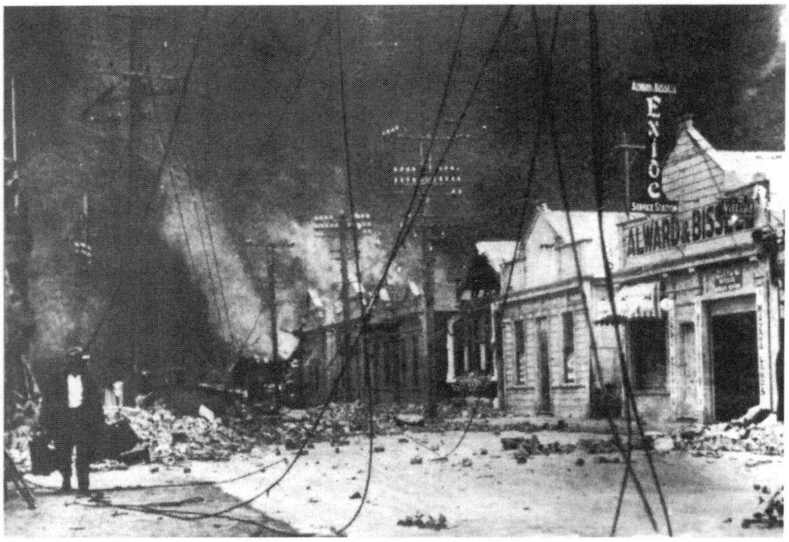

Tennyson Street, Napier. Fires burn out of control following the 1931 earthquake. (Alexander Turnbull Library, Ref: PAColl-6585-77)

The generosity of fellow New Zealanders was profound. Temporary homes were offered by people within a reasonable distance of the quake zone. Palmerston North was particularly sympathetic, offering to take in 5000 evacuees.

When it was first reported that a major earthquake had struck Napier, Hastings and nearby Hawke's Bay towns, newspaper reporters were dispatched to cover the story. One of the first reporters to reach the earthquake area approached through Waipukurau, Waipawa and Te Aute, heading north towards the major centres of Hawke's Bay. The famous Te Aute College was badly damaged and there was evidence of the quake along the road. The destruction in the business centre of Hastings was bad enough, yet all the while the reporter was conscious of an eerie, ominous red glow as he approached Napier, the largest city. He found that Hastings was horrifying but Napier was considerably worse. Going from Waipukurau to Napier was like descending into hell.

Communication among the survivors was a problem in the early days after the earthquake. Rumours spread almost as rapidly as the fires, which in Napier swept through ten acres of buildings before they burnt out. One story on the broken streets of Napier was that both Auckland and Wellington had borne the brunt of a series of massive, far-flung earthquakes. Such speculation may have provided some strange comfort to the Hawke's Bay survivors – the fact that they weren't in this alone. With newspaper offices knocked out by the quake, there was no way to keep the people abreast of developments.

No news may have been good news as survivors continued searching the wrecked buildings for possible survivors. Ongoing earthquake aftershocks remained a problem, and several searchers lost their lives when weakened walls and façades collapsed on top of them. It was a telling statistic when it was gauged that over three-fifths of the dead were crushed on pavements or while running out of disintegrating buildings.

The death toll from the quake was officially recorded at 256.

The death toll from the quake was officially recorded at 256. In Napier 161 died. Hastings recorded 93, most of whom lost their lives in department stores and the public library. In the town of Wairoa to the north, two residents died. Over the years the exact number of deaths has been questioned. This situation resulted from cases like the old man who was injured and transferred to Wellington Hospital, where he died. He was buried in Karori Cemetery without a headstone and his name was not added to the earthquake memorial. Nor was it added to the official death toll. There may be other examples of this kind, along with the case of the premature birth and subsequent death of twins in the quake zone, with the double tragedy being attributed to the extreme trauma experienced by the babies' mother.

As much as the Hawke's Bay quake affected the lives of survivors in a profound way, the physical landscape was much changed too. Hillsides collapsed into valleys, often blocking or changing the course of rivers and streams. Some rivers changed their course simply because of the upheaval of river beds. Terrifying fissures opened up the land, trees were uprooted and well-known landmarks disappeared. New landmarks emerged. An area of 300 acres was sheared off completely from its former coastal location and became a promontory jutting into the ocean.

Perhaps the most dramatic effect the quake had on the local landscape was the emergence of the up-thrust sea bed of the Ahuriri Lagoon. Eventually 9000 acres of new farmland would replace the lagoon, although for many years the salt content of the soil presented problems. The old Ahuriri Lagoon would eventually produce healthy pasture and crops, in a place where yachts used to sail and children swam.

The destruction of the business section of Napier was so complete that when the time came to rebuild the city, something unique emerged. The city was reconstructed in the art deco style of architecture, lending the new Napier a distinctive appearance, so much so that Napier's art deco buildings and fixtures now attract thousands of visitors and tourists. Had the 1931 earthquake not occurred, this development would not have come about. But what a price to pay.

13

A WALL OF WATER

The Kopuawhara flash flood 1938

The Kopuawhara stream was usually a gurgling, inconsequential watercourse, on the banks of which a temporary settlement known as Kopuawhara No 4 Public Works camp had been erected to house railway construction workers building the Napier–Gisborne railway line. The stream provided drinking and washing water for the camp and somewhere for hot and tired construction workers to wallow in the cool shallows following a hard day's labour.

It seemed an ideal place to set up a temporary settlement as the railway line advanced. It had been of little consequence when the weather patterns of the area were considered. The Gisborne region was subject to sudden rainstorms that could often see watercourses become raging torrents. On the night of 18 February 1938 a huge cloudburst in the hills around the camp affected the Kopuawhara stream in this very way. The build-up of water was phenomenal. Soon it became apparent that people living close to the streams in the area would have flood waters to deal with.

The lines of huts and tents that made up the Kopuawhara camp housed 47 workers. The camp also contained a dining room, cookhouse, bathhouse and blacksmith's shop. Kopuawhara No 4 camp was one of four such settlements in the vicinity which housed hundreds of men, women and children. The No 4 camp was designated for single men. Ominously it was located close to the stream.

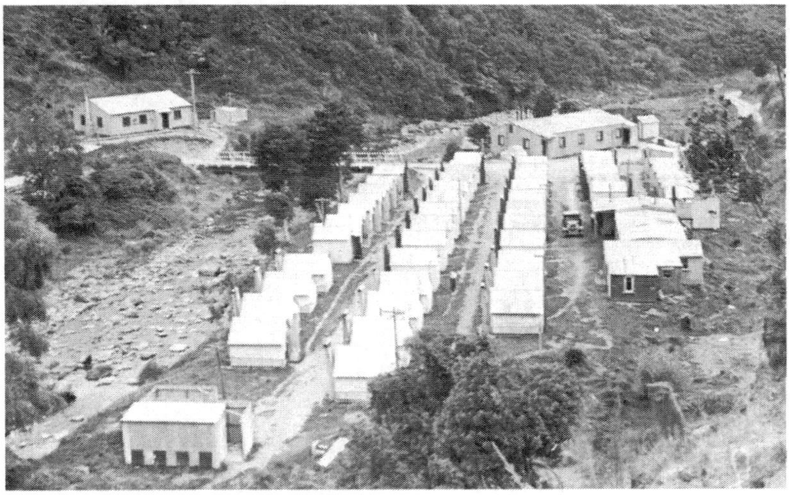

Before and after. The Kopuawhara No 4 public works camp before the flood-and almost totally destroyed after the stream became a torrent.
(Alexander Turnbull Library, Ref: PAColl-4431-02 and PAColl-4431-01)

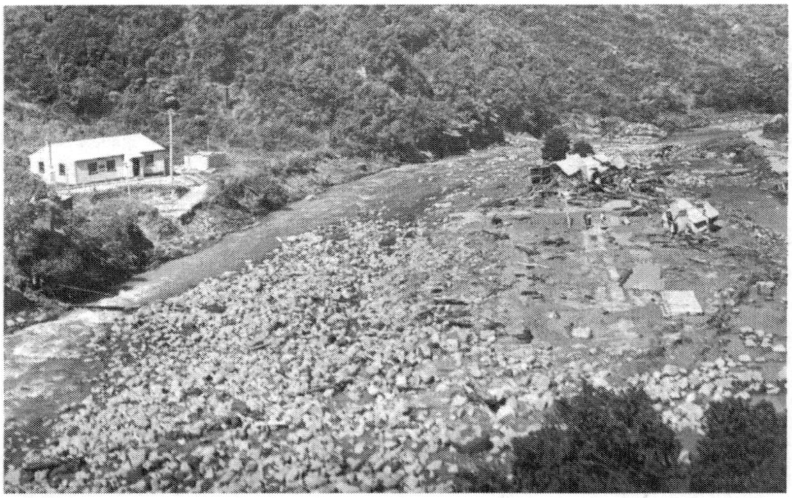

Heroes invariably emerge from disastrous situations. At Kopuawhara the hero was a railway construction worker named Ted Tracey. He was not sleeping well, a result of the basic, hard mattress on his bunk. It was said that because the workmen in the camp were enthusiastic workers – only too pleased to go the extra mile in years when unemployment was rife – they usually collapsed into bed in a fatigued state. They could sleep on anything.

On the night of 18 February 1938, Ted Tracey tossed and turned on his hard mattress. Perhaps his sleep patterns were also disturbed by premonitions, or perhaps he was just a poor sleeper. If so, it was just as well. At 3.30 in the morning he woke with a start. He had already heard the cloudburst and the driving rain, but now a different sound filled him with horror.

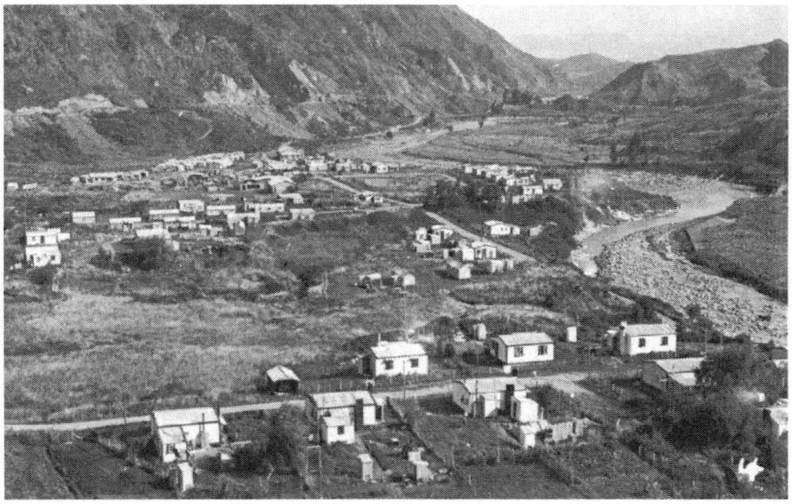

The Kopuawhara No 3 Camp, situated nearby, emerged from the flood largely unscathed. (Alexander Turnbull Library, Ref: PAColl-4431-03)

The sound of a roaring flash flood drove Ted Tracey from his bed. The turbulent waters were in the process of breaching the stream's banks and water was surging through those huts located closest to the watercourse. Tracey could have sought his own salvation by running across the footbridge over the stream towards higher ground, but his prime concern was for the safety of his fellow workmates. With considerable initiative he made it to the camp cookhouse, grabbed the dinner gong and began beating it frantically in an attempt to wake those still sleeping in their bunks. Most were unaware of the danger posed by the rapidly rising waters; others heard the gong and thought it was some drunken oaf on the rampage.

Eventually Tracey gave up on the gong and waded from hut to hut bashing on doors. He was also aware that his foreman, who was hard of hearing, needed a more immediate summons. Tracey smashed his way into the foreman's hut and assisted him to safety. Tracey thought nothing of his own welfare as he continued to alert and assist his workmates. The following day, when the full horror of the situation became evident, his body was found some five kilometres downstream.

A five-metre-high wall of water hit the camp as Ted Tracey did his rounds.

A five-metre-high wall of water hit the camp as Ted Tracey did his rounds. A bridge was wrecked by rocks and logs, propelled by a water surge reckoned to be flowing at close to 40 miles per hour. The majority of the huts and tents were levelled and swept away by the flood. Some workers were taken out by the waters. Some probably drowned in their sleep. Others, awake to possibilities, climbed onto a large work truck which appeared to be a solid bulwark. The truck was no match for the force of the flood. It toppled over and all eleven men who had sought sanctuary were drowned. The bonnet of the truck was found 12 kilometres downstream. No fragments of the rest of the truck were ever found.

There were other tales of gallantry. One man, aware that the camp waitress was probably trapped in her quarters behind the cookhouse, set out to rescue her. He subsequently lost his life while trying to reach her. It was later considered likely that the waitress, the only woman to die in the maelstrom, was probably one of the first victims. Her hut had disappeared early in the piece.

The young daughter of the camp caterer survived through the efforts of an elderly man who held the child above the flood waters until the torrent had subsided a little. The caterer's 17year-old son showed considerable initiative by grasping and pulling a man into a hut, away from the danger of the torrent.

At first light the search began for victims. Communications had been compromised, not only in the immediate district, but to the rest of the country as well. Eventually police parties from nearby towns made it over damaged roads to the Kopuawhara Valley and the doomed campsite. Bodies were found over a vast area, often located in ruined farmland now smothered in deep layers of silt, mud and upstream debris. Objects from the camp were found miles downstream. And bodies. Eventually the death toll was set at 21, although there were fears that some bodies may have been buried under the silt or, like the thousands of sheep and cattle, washed out to sea. But for the bravery of Ted Tracey and others, the toll would have been much greater. In addition, another public works camp had been in the path of the flood five kilometres downstream.

The second camp housed 47 people and was devastated by the flash flood, but not one occupant lost his life. One of them was awoken at 3.30a.m., roused by a power failure that he noticed when a light left on by his sleeping companion had cut out. The heavy rain concerned the man and when he noticed water seeping in under the door, he investigated the situation. As the water rose, the alarm was raised and everyone made it to higher ground. It was a near thing. Five minutes later the water was waist deep and would have condemned numerous workmen to a watery grave.

It was said with sadness that the rest of New Zealand often only got to know the location of backwaters like Kopuawhara when tragedies of this kind occurred. And then it was often some time after the event. Six months later, farmers in the Kopuawhara Valley were still dealing with a sea of silt and mud. Two thousand acres were affected and half of that was still submerged. The February cloudburst was bad enough, but further flooding hit the area in April.

Michael Savage, the New Zealand Prime Minister, described the disaster as 'a phenomenal visitation'. He declared the causes as being entirely beyond human control, that no wisdom or foresight could have prevented the disaster. Doubts remain, however, about the placement of the devastated camp so close to a watercourse in a storm-prone area – irrespective of its temporary nature.

14

OUT OF MIND, OUT OF SIGHT

The Seacliff fire 1942

During the era when the Seacliff fire struck, ordinary Kiwis were as far away from a compassionate and intelligent appraisal of insanity and mental health as earlier generations had been. We weren't quite treating the afflicted in some imitation of the medieval Bedlam, but our tendency to turn our backs on the mentally ill was equally judgemental. 'Out of mind, out of sight' might have been the modus operandi for New Zealand in 1942.

If you were out of your mind, you could expect to end up in one of the gothic brick institutions situated in lonely recesses of the new land. These establishments were off the beaten track, miles from anywhere, cast adrift in rural landscapes where normal folk did not have to be reminded of the plight of the mentally afflicted. It was best for them to be incarcerated. The poor souls would find succour and companionship in the forbidding ramparts of mental institutions, miles from the mainstream where normal people went about their business.

In those days New Zealanders were terrified of mental illness. If one of your family had to go down south for a while, or up the line, or out east eventually – all euphemisms referencing the committal of someone to a gothic psychiatric hospital – it was a great shame and stigma. People whispered behind hands about such awful things. Affected family members were told very little. Schizophrenia and other kinds of mental illness carried unpronounceable names that you would not want to enunciate anyway.

The reason for the fear was that people had heard all sorts of rumours about 'loony bins'. Unfortunately they were often true. Before effective medication became available, doctors often used electroconvulsive therapy (ECT) and straightjackets when things got really bad. As the years passed, many patients became institutionalised. There was no cure. They could not survive in Main Street or even on the fringes. And yet Janet Frame, one of New Zealand's most famous authors, spent several years in such a place before achieving success in the wider world. That place was Seacliff Hospital, near Dunedin.

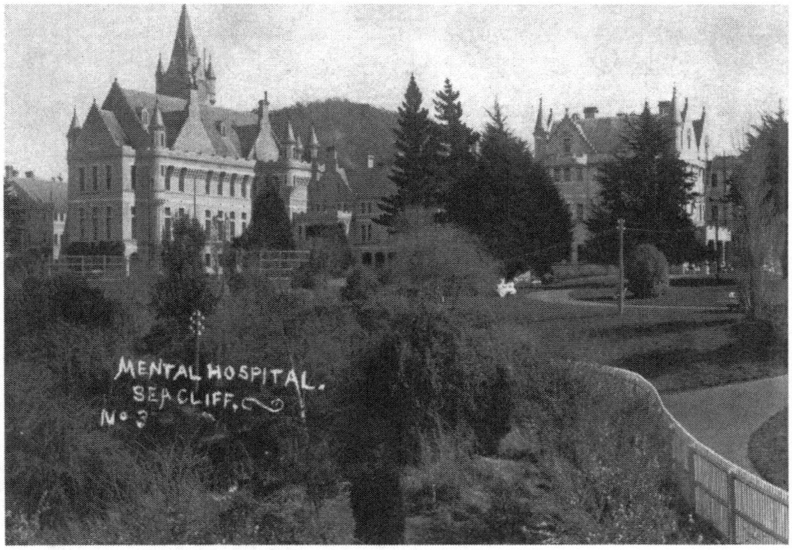

The lofty towers of Seacliff Hospital in its heyday. (Alexander Turnbull Library, Ref: PAColl-8769-02)

When Seacliff Hospital was built in the late nineteenth century, it was the largest building in New Zealand. It was designed by surveyor Robert Lawson and had many extravagant features. Built in the gothic style, it boasted many turrets, a tower, a spire and a gabled roof and presented a grand façade to the world. Over the years, it became the epitome of the 'gothic institution' that came to be associated with mental hospitals throughout the country.

Although it was a massive place, accommodating 500 patients and 50 staff, it was flawed from the outset. Surveyor Lawson was made aware early on that the land on which Seacliff was built was prone to land movements and slips. The construction of the hospital continued unabated and the building was finally opened in 1884.

Institutions like Seacliff had a good reputation for confinement and care. Confinement consisted of ensuring that all patients were securely contained. That, for many in 1942, was enough. In keeping with the 'out of sight, out of mind' mindset of 'normal' New Zealanders, Seacliff provided the safe confinement of patients that society required for over fifty years. Then, on the evening of 8 December 1942, a fire broke out in Ward 5, a women's only ward. The fire quickly took hold.

It would have been a horrific scene that greeted members of the Seacliff Mental Hospital fire brigade, as they set about dealing with their biggest challenge. Flames were shooting out savagely from the roof of Ward 5. The front section of the ward was in a state of collapse and it was palpably obvious that few could have survived such a conflagration.

Flames were shooting out savagely from the roof of Ward 5.

Nurses and attendants concentrated on evacuating nearby female wards at the northern end of the burning ward. Firemen, aware of the futility of fighting the Ward 5 fire, turned their attention to saving the main building, from which all the patients were evacuated and transferred to the nurses' home and the recreation hall.

Attempts to fight the Ward 5 fire and save the patients seemed to have been largely waived early in the piece. Admittedly, firemen tried to break into the burning building through a south-facing door, but the flames drove them back. And of course those trapped inside were unable to get out because, as this was a mental hospital, none of the doors could be opened or unlocked from the inside. When some of the patients tried to escape through the windows they found them barred by wooden shutters. Windows on the other side of the building were sealed by wire gratings.

Many considered the ward a death trap. There was an uneasy trade-off between patient safety and public safety. After all, most of the patients were regarded as a menace to the general public, to themselves and to An obvious possible cause was that of arson. other patients. The attitudes of the times dictated that public safety held precedence and for that reason Ward 5 patients were locked in from the outside.

The scenes and sounds as Ward 5 went up in flames must have been like something out of Bedlam. The screams didn't last for long. The fire burnt like a firestorm, with a strong southerly fanning the flames. It was almost a gale at times, and the fire became so fierce that it could be seen from the township of Palmerston, nearly twenty miles away. Ward 5 was a wooden building and in no time it became an inferno.

Thirty-seven patients out of 39 died in the fire. The attrition rate was horrifying, although over the years hospital staff had communicated their fears of what might happen if Ward 5 ever caught alight. Despite the hardnosed attitudes of hospital administrators and some nurses and attendants, the patients' welfare was of concern to some. In fact, at the height of the fire several acts of heroism shone through.

Arthur Driscoll, the hospital fire-brigade leader realised there was one window that had still not been surrounded by fire. He prised the wire grating off with a hatchet and was able to assist a patient through the window. Her nightdress was burning but he successfully staunched the flames. Although suffering from burns, she was one of the two survivors. The other was a patient who found a way to the second storey, where she was able to use a fire escape and scramble to safety. It is considered likely that neither the location – nor even the existence – of the second-storey fire escapes would have been general knowledge. And in their panic-stricken state it was thought unlikely that most would have stopped to consider this option.

The fire was one of the most ferocious in New Zealand's history. The blaze was first discovered around 10p.m., yet in under an hour the ward had basically disappeared, along with 37 souls. What remained was a tragic tangle of twisted iron bedsteads and buckled roofing iron.

Much of the story of the Seacliff Mental Hospital fire relates to finding the cause of the blaze. A Commission of Enquiry was set up and a great deal of evidence paraded. An obvious possible cause was that of arson. It was simple enough to declare that a patient had somehow set the fire and enquire no further, but the commission was not presented with any evidence to support this. Another possible cause, however, was debated at length.

An obvious possible cause was that of arson.

The hospital was located on land that sloped down to the Pacific Ocean. It was an unusual setting, and from its early days there were those who considered it possible that landslides could disturb the mainly brick buildings. In fact there had been earth movements in the area and the hospital was affected. The link between this situation and the fire came from the likelihood that electric lighting installation wires could have crossed as the earth and buildings moved. This could have set off a fire.

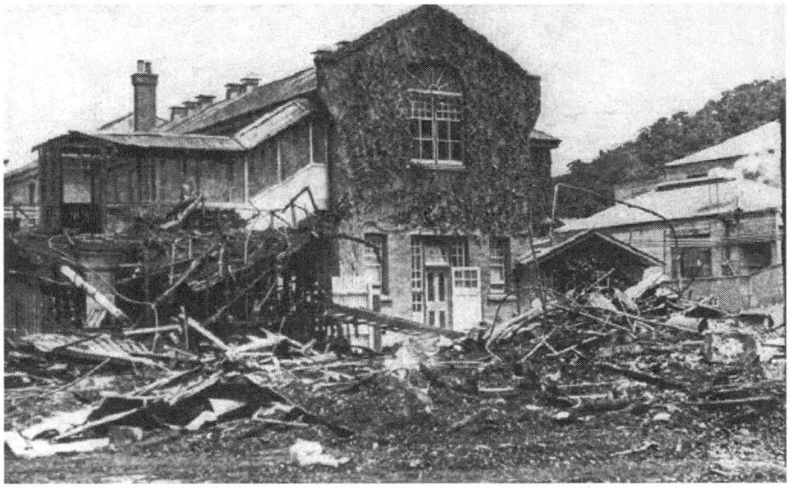

The ruins of Ward 5 after the catastrophic fire. (Alexander Turnbull Library/New Zealand Herald)

Ward 5 was located on the part of the Seacliff property that was the most unstable. This had been known for years, but the long-term danger that could be caused by such earth movements was swept under the carpet. Two years before the fire, the authorities had acted on this knowledge and taken steps to jack up one end of Ward 5 a full two feet to strengthen that end of the building.

Some years earlier, three wards had been physically removed because of the land slipping. There had also been a suspicious fire in a female ward that destroyed a dining room. The cause was never ascertained. Perhaps the crossing of electrical wires as a result of buildings moving had already occurred.

Another possible explanation put forward was rats nibbling through wires, but because there was no evidence of this the Commission of Enquiry did not feel justified in accepting it as a likely cause.

However, the commission did declare Ward 5 to have been dangerous in terms of fire hazards. The design of the building was such that if fire did break out there would be little to prevent an escalation. For a start, it was wooden. While newer sections of the hospital had been fitted with automatic fire alarms, Ward 5's alarm involved the unlocking of a cabinet and the pushing of a button. Valuable seconds would be lost in activating such a device, and what would happen if staff were unable to access and activate the fire alarm because it was already cut off by flames?

The commission also recommended the installation of sprinkler systems in all mental hospitals. They gave a more general ruling that when it was necessary to lock patients in individual rooms by securing doors and window shutters, it should be feasible to provide each room with an emergency exit that could be accessed from the outside.

The commission further suggested that institutions should employ an officer in charge of the fire brigades (where one hadn't been appointed), and provide modern rescue equipment.

The Seacliff fire of 1942 remained New Zealand's worst fire in terms of loss of life until Christchurch's Ballantynes fire in 1947, which resulted in 41 deaths. Seacliff Hospital has long gone: it finally closed in 1973. Most of the buildings have been demolished or removed from a site they should never really have occupied in the first place. Much of the land has reverted to woodland and private ownership. Several of the smaller hospital buildings have been renovated and now operate as private dwellings.

Seacliff Hospital was magnificently situated. From the site today you can look down on the wide Pacific, while listening to the distant roar of the ocean and the wind in the resurgent trees. Those are the only sounds, apart from cars and the occasional clatter of passing trains on the main line that used to bring patients to Seacliff. The screams and the clamour have gone. Nearly 100 years of incarceration, and an hour's incineration in 1942, are horrible memories that belong to another era.

15

TOO MUCH SPEED

The Hyde rail accident 1943

It happens on our highways too. The advent of a long weekend sees hundreds heading for leisure destinations and special events being held at the end of the yellow brick road – or New Zealand's often challenging highways. People longing to get away from their usual humdrum lives but not wishing to be snarled up in traffic jams get in their cars and put the foot down. Speed and crowded highways on the eve of precious long weekends can see our road toll climb. Many hundreds of New Zealanders have lost their lives on Fridays preceding long weekends.

It happened to a train once: the daily passenger express from Cromwell to Dunedin in 1943. The long King's Birthday weekend was approaching and, in the middle of a wretched winter and with World War Two raging, Central Otago folk were anxious to get to the city, where minds could be temporarily taken off the harshness of life. Not that the passengers had any control over the speed of the train. But you had to consider the motivation of the train driver who was doing his best to reach Dunedin in as short a time as possible.

Speed was the overriding factor experienced by passengers on the Central Otago Express as it roared down the track beyond the small town of Hyde. A certain amount of swaying was a feature of many New Zealand train journeys, but this was different. Suitcases, bags and other luggage were jostled out of the racks and fell to the floor. Passengers were losing their footing in the aisles as they shuffled around to retrieve the luggage. Regular travellers on the express felt something was not right. One man who had left his seat to talk to friends in another carriage cut short his socialising when he found it almost impossible to stand. Normally the express didn't go this fast.

The daily Cromwell to Dunedin express was introduced in 1936, replacing a thrice-weekly express that had been supported by mixed trains made up of goods wagons and one or two passenger carriages. The mixed train was described as being as 'slow as a wet week', so there was general approval when the new service in 1936 was inaugurated to operate on a daily basis. Mind you, on 4 June 1943, the slow pace of the mixed train would have been welcomed by passengers on the express as it hurtled along south of Hyde. AB 782, the engine at the head of the train, was certainly earning its keep. The seven passenger carriages, guard's van and two wagons of freight seemed a doddle. There were 113 passengers on board, an increase in patronage because of the looming long weekend. Despite the heavy load the engine continued speeding.

At the outset, in 1936, the express was tabled to depart Cromwell at 9a.m. and reach Dunedin at 5.20p.m. This schedule was advanced by half an hour in 1937, and although the adjustment led to faster running, it didn't account for the hectic speed that June day as the train headed towards the winter show and horse racing at Wingatui and all the other pleasures that a long weekend in Dunedin could bring.

On a winter's afternoon in Central Otago, a farmer was working in his fields, wondering if the banking clouds would lead to sleet or worse, snow overnight. With the war raging, the farmer momentarily pondered his position in a quiet backwater of peaceful New Zealand with little more to worry about than the winter weather. His idle thoughts were suddenly interrupted by a terrible crashing sound coming from the railway cutting not far from his property.

The Cromwell to Dunedin express was due, and the farmer was hoping that the crash had nothing to do with the most famous of Central Otago's trains. When he reached the deep cutting carrying the railway line, the farmer was confronted by a hellish scene. What lay before him was New Zealand's worst railway accident to date. Twenty-one passengers were killed and 47 injured.

What lay before him was New Zealand's worst railway accident to date.

As the farmer was assailed by screams and groans, it was obvious that many passengers were trapped in the huge amount of wreckage that clogged the rail cutting. Instinctively he ran a mile to telephone for assistance before returning to the ghastly scene. It was only then that he began searching through the mangled carriages for survivors – including, he hoped, his son. Help took an interminable time to arrive, but when it did the farmer had already found his son's broken body. He had died instantly. There was a sad twist to the discovery, because his son, returning to army camp, had had to clap on the pace to catch the train at the last station.

It was reckoned that the train was travelling at 110 kph as it approached the critical curve. The speed limit on the corner was 48 kph.

The express, through excessive speed, failed to negotiate the 183-metre radius curve in a deep cutting known as Straw Cutting. This occurred not long after it had crossed Six Mile Creek, located between Hyde and Rock and Pillar. The train derailed with the engine ending up jammed against the cutting bank. It was approximately 60 metres from where it left the line. The concussion of the crash led to the boiler exploding which, if nothing else, led to the dousing of the engine fire. Had the fire continued burning there was a good chance it would have ignited the carriages that also left the tracks. Unfortunately, the boiler explosion led to the serious scalding of the express fireman.

All seven carriages left the track. Only the guard's van and two goods wagons at the rear of the train stayed on the line. Four of the carriages telescoped together, causing terrible injuries to the passengers. The second carriage flipped over and ended up in front of the engine. Such was the force of the crash that the bogies and underpinning of one carriage were wrenched into an S shape.

All seven carriages left the track.

One of the much-lauded characteristics of Central Otago is its wild beauty and remoteness. The same remote nature of the region was soon to prove a bugbear for rescue workers and medical staff. It took these Good Samaritans an hour and a half to finally reach the accident site. Reports of the accident had reached the town of Middlemarch but the seriousness of the crash had somehow been played down. The received wisdom was that there were possibly a few injuries, and as a consequence medical staff showed less urgency than they might have. However, once they caught a glimpse of the wreck from the road, they realised they would be dealing with a major incident.

As word spread to outlying areas, the people of Central Otago rallied. A pub owner sent mattresses, blankets, sheets, first-aid equipment, brandy and whisky by horseback. One of the first doctors on the scene described the situation as resembling the aftermath of a bomb blast. Splintered wood from the carriages, bent steel and the remains of seats clogged the cutting and littered the surrounding paddocks.

The carriages at the rear of the train were relatively unscathed and several passengers who were not injured helped, as best they could, to look after those worst affected. Some passengers were trapped in the wreckage for hours.

Eventually the dead and injured were transferred to morgue and hospital, the rescue teams, medical staff and railway maintenance crews finished their sad and often grisly tasks, and the country surrounding Straw Cutting fell silent again. However, the disaster affected just about everyone living in the Maniototo region, where the crash site was located.

Reports of the accident emerged. There were good- and bad-luck stories. Sometimes there were both. An elderly woman survived but lost her husband, daughter and two grandchildren. A baby was found unharmed in its bassinet deep in the debris. One woman who survived had relinquished her seat to a mother and baby not long before the crash occurred. The mother and baby were killed.

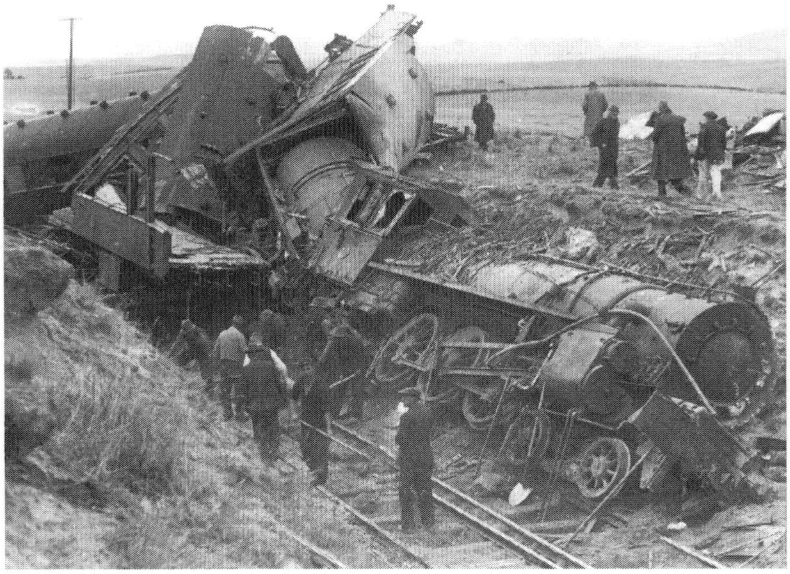

Carnage at Hyde. Workmen were faced with a huge task following the disaster, (Otago Daily Times)

Fate also played its hand in the case of a family who regularly travelled on the express to attend the show in Dunedin at King's Birthday weekend and regularly booked their accommodation for the following year's events while paying for the current one. For some reason they had cancelled their booking on the very morning of the fateful crash.

The driver and fireman both survived. The driver injured his arm and both he and the fireman suffered scalding when the engine boiler burst.

Inevitably, it seemed, the Board of Enquiry into the crash found that speed was the overriding factor. The train was travelling at over twice the stipulated speed when it attempted to round Straw Cutting. Simple centrifugal force caused it to derail in spectacular fashion. All eyes turned to the driver, 55-year-old John Corcoran. Accusations of dereliction of duty were staring him in the face. But why the extreme speed? It was true that most on board couldn't wait to get to the bright lights of Dunedin, but not at the expense of safety.

Corcoran was deemed to have been drunk at the controls of the train. Empty beer bottles were found in the vicinity of the engine's cab. Had the pressure of overwork and continuous shifts got to him? Obviously that was no excuse, but during the war years workers in general were stretched to the limit. With so many men of working age committed to the war effort, there were fewer left behind to man 'essential services'.

What were the responsibilities of the fireman and guard regarding the state of the driver? Had they been drinking too? And what about the stationmaster and other rail officials at the station before Hyde? Stories began circulating about evidence of drinking before the train even reached Hyde. One observer who saw the train pass through Kokonga, the last station before Hyde, was of the opinion that the crew members had obviously been drinking. So were the guard and fireman slurping turps as well?

It was also observed that there was obvious reluctance on the part of the stationmaster, as far back as Waipiata, to have rescuers heading south to the crash site to offer help. He may have noticed the crew's condition and now, despite the seriousness of the crash, felt the need to protect them. Perhaps this was one of the reasons the rescue teams took so long to get to the accident site.

Attitudes towards alcohol during the war, and after it, were tolerant, even in workplace situations. If the practice was well masked and fellow-workers turned a blind eye, what did it really matter if dirty, hot, thirsty work like driving a steam engine was lubricated by a beer or two? It seems extraordinary in this day and age, but drinking and engine-driving were not an uncommon combination.

He was found guilty and sentenced to three years' jail.

Perhaps the driver had nodded off, the result of too little sleep and too much beer. Whatever the precise reason, he was found to be impaired. He was later tried at the Dunedin Supreme Court on a charge of manslaughter. He was found guilty and sentenced to three years' jail. The guard was reprimanded for not taking action at the train's breakneck speed, but he was not criminally prosecuted.

Thoughts were expressed that perhaps the train had been rollicking around Straw Cutting at excessive speed for years, but on this occasion the speed climbed too high. The government of the day became liable for compensation claims once the driver had been charged.

Time passes and trends change. And while hard history may fade, it will never die. Younger – and older – generations have taken the Otago Rail Trail to their hearts. Much of the section of the old Central Otago railway line that was closed in 1990 was soon converted into a modern, interactive phenomenon called a rail trail. It was a masterfully simple way of creating something for tourists to call their own. Tourist developers took to the idea of converting the ancient bridges, viaducts, tunnels, embankments and cuttings of a closed railway line into something tourists could cycle, run or walk along, witnessing the same stellar scenery that train riders enjoyed once upon a time, but doing it independently, at their own pace and without having to be herded like sheep into carriages and told that the train would be leaving at exactly 9.00a.m. All aboard! Do as you are told.

The beauty of the rail trail was that the hard construction and clearing work had already been done. It was just a matter of smoothing over the rough bits and filling in a few gaps, so that runners, walkers, cyclists and even horse riders could retrace the route of the old trains. The Otago Rail Trail follows the path of the Central Otago Express that ran on 4 June 1943. When runners or cyclists negotiate a 183-metre radius curve in a deep cutting once known as Straw Cutting – not long after crossing Six Mile Creek, between the town of Hyde and Rock and Pillar – they are covering the ground that was covered in blood when the Central Otago Express left the line in 1943.

It probably doesn't mean much to most people any more, but there have been reports of modern travellers pausing at the spot where the AB engine and seven carriages derailed and 21 innocent people died.

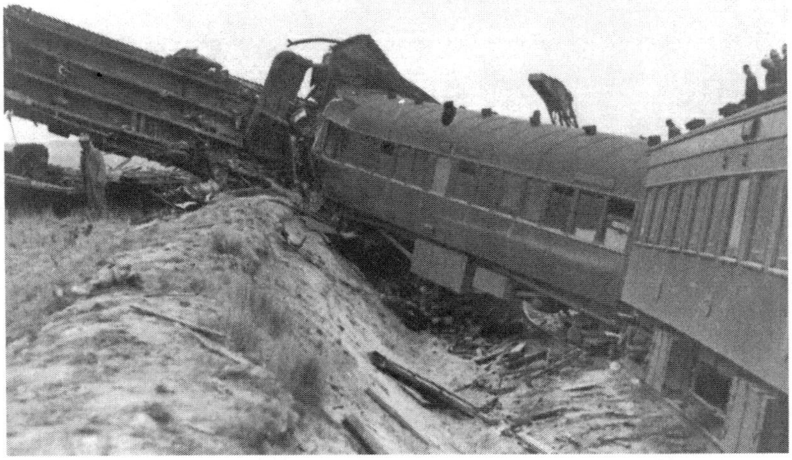

Carriages were thrown off the tracks as a result of excessive speed. [Otago Daily Times)

A memorial cairn to those who lost their lives in the Hyde railway disaster of 1943 was dedicated on 17 February 1991. The location of the cairn is roughly 500 metres south of the site of the crash, beside State Highway 87. That it took so long for the memorial to be erected, and the deceased to be honoured, speaks volumes of the disaster being a victim of wartime restrictions on information being disseminated to the population.

The isolation of the accident site on a secondary line, miles from anywhere and at a time when New Zealanders in general had their minds set on World

War Two, meant the event flew under the radar at the time and even in later years. Little news of the disaster was circulated to the population at large. Relatives of victims did not receive word of their tragic losses until the day after the disaster.

When the memorial to the victims of 1953's Tangiwai disaster was established, relatives and friends of victims of the Hyde disaster began working towards a memorial relating to 1943's sad event. The memorial cairn is the result.

16

THE SECRET CRASH

The crash of USAF Liberator at Whenuapai 1943

When Japan entered World War Two on 7 December 1941, it plunged New Zealand into a state of terror. Marching steadily south through nation after nation inflicting hideous cruelty on its captives, Japan clearly had its sights set firmly on the country. Young men who had been following the war in Europe from the safety of a newspaper were compelled to enlist with all speed.

In the six months following the Pearl Harbor attack it was widely believed that a Japanese invasion of New Zealand could occur at any time within the next 24 hours. Some fathers later confessed that they were planning to shoot their wives and daughters rather than let them fall into Japanese hands. Japanese nationals living in New Zealand at the commencement of hostilities were interned in camps.

But the situation changed on 12 June 1942 when large numbers of American servicemen arrived in Auckland and Wellington, brought here partly for rest and recreation and partly for strategic military purposes.

War matériel stockpiles and the presence of huge American aircraft and ships presented an enormous morale-boosting spectacle. Fathers could now sleep at night rather than lie awake expecting the sirens to start at any moment.

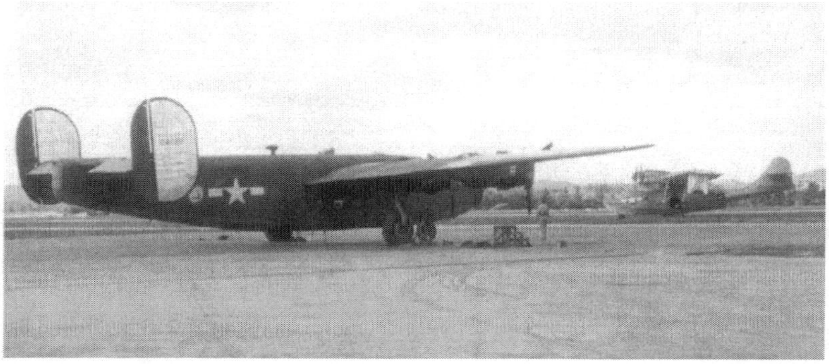

A C-87A Liberator Express of the same type that crashed at Whenuapai in 1943. (Air Force Museum of New Zealand, Wigram)

Auckland's international airport was at Whenuapai, which was host to many arriving US planes. A frequent visitor to Whenuapai throughout the war years was the lumbering B-24 Liberator aircraft, and later the C-87 Liberator Express, which ferried men and supplies to US bases in the Pacific. The enormous need for aircraft and crews in the Pacific led to four US civilian airlines operating Liberators under contract to Air Transport Command.

The C-87 harboured many technical faults and was not popular with air crews, who coped with engine fires and typically flew on with fuel leaking throughout the aircraft. The Liberator became known as the flying coffin. One fact that emerged after the war was that more aircraft were lost in accidents than were lost in combat. Shortly before the Americans arrived, on 9 June 1942, a Flying Fortress laden with bombs crashed on take-off, setting off enormous explosions in the middle of the night, leading many terrified Aucklanders to believe the feared Japanese invasion had begun. To avoid public alarm, much adverse war news was kept from the general population, so it was over a year before it was confirmed that 11 visiting airmen had been killed that night.

But more secrecy surrounded the crash of a US C-87 Liberator at 2.30a.m. on 2 August 1943. It was many years after the war before the facts started to seep out. Writing in 1998, J. W. Sim of Alexandra recalled that he was on his way to work at Whenuapai in the middle of the night when he saw a Liberator which had just taken off. The left wing was down and the aircraft kept banking more and more to the left, with flames apparently coming from one of the left wing engines. The plane began disintegrating as it crashed in a mangrove swamp and caught fire.

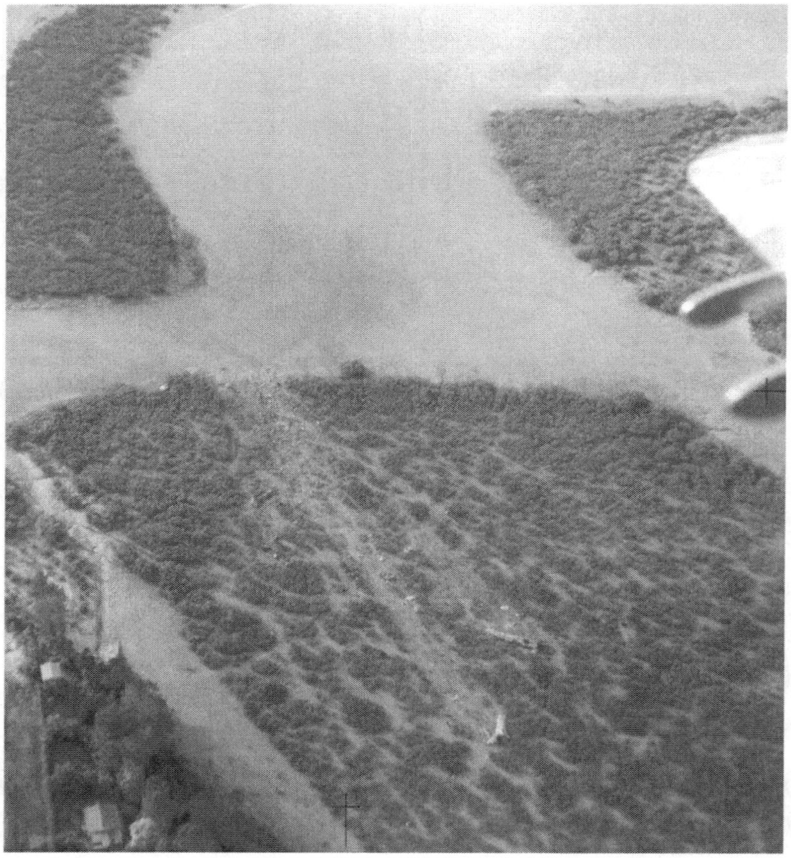

An aerial view of the crash scene, with some wreckage still visible, (Air Force Museum of New Zealand, Wigram)

Rumours spread that there were no survivors, but it was generally known around the air base that some Japanese officials were on board and there were confused stories about a prisoner exchange. Such was the secrecy of the mission, the pilots had no idea who was on board or how many people were in the passenger compartment behind them. In fact, there were 22 Japanese men, women and children, three Thais and five crew, and 570 kg of mail destined for Queensland, en route to New Guinea. There the passengers were to be part of a negotiated exchange in which some Allied prisoners would be released. Out of 30 persons on board, 14 were killed – the worst death toll in New Zealand aviation history at that time. The Liberator was under a United Airlines civilian air crew, with Captain Herschel Laughlin at the controls and John Wisda as co-pilot. Wisda continued his career in aviation after the war, and many years later flew a Boeing 747 for United Airlines. It was at this time that he gave an interview with his recollections of the Liberator crash, before passing away in 2004.

Such was the secrecy of the mission, the pilots had no idea who was on board.

Wisda recalled that the pilots and crew had been working continuously for 26 days ferrying personnel to and from Guadalcanal. On 1 August 1943, he had not long collapsed exhausted into bed when he was woken at 10p.m. with a telephone call to take a special trip out at midnight. 'It was raining quite hard, foggy and cold. It was not exactly a night you wanted to be flying aeroplanes but they said this had to go, so off we went,' recalled Wisda. The passengers boarded while the pilots were doing their checks, with young children sitting on their mothers' laps. They were not ready to take off until well after midnight.

The air traffic controller, Pilot Officer P. Stephenson, recalled that the Liberator, identified only as JD4, took off on a northbound runway with a full length of gooseneck flares, but conditions were poor, visibility was just two and a half miles with heavy cloud cover, and there was a brisk northerly wind with rain. The aircraft became airborne halfway down the runway opposite the control tower, then climbed fairly steeply with its landing lights switched off, and seemed to be climbing normally with the navigation lights on. At approximately 600 feet the aircraft turned quite steeply to the left, continued for a short period then began to lose height. Perceiving disaster, Stephenson called the fire tender and ambulance to start moving, moments before a great flash of light showed the aircraft's fate.

With everything pitch black outside, Wisda had sensed that things were not right as the left wing seemed low, and argued with Laughlin who insisted the gyroscope still showed the wings to be level. Wisda convinced his captain that he should turn on the left engine turbo charger to level the wings, but it was too late and the Liberator crashed heavily on its belly into a mangrove swamp and caught fire. Eight Japanese and three Thai passengers were killed, along with three of the five crew. A 300-metre trail of debris led rescuers to Wisda, badly cut and bruised, taking refuge next to a burning tyre to keep warm. He was the last survivor to be picked up. It took surgeons 13 hours to clean mud from his wounds. But the cause of the accident was put down to pilot fatigue leading to the omission of some vital cockpit checks – in particular the gyroscope, which was still locked.

It was feared the Japanese might believe the deaths were deliberate and take reprisals against Allied prisoners, or alternatively that the disaster would invoke a direct attack. Thus a strict cloak of secrecy was laid down. As late as 2015, access to archival files relating to the Japanese internees was still restricted. The official USAF accident report lists full names and occupations of the Japanese occupants, indicating many were families, with occupations such as male clerk, male director, male student or fisherman. They were consular staff members and their families, together with employees of a Japanese merchant company who had been held as aliens and moved from Tonga in 1941.

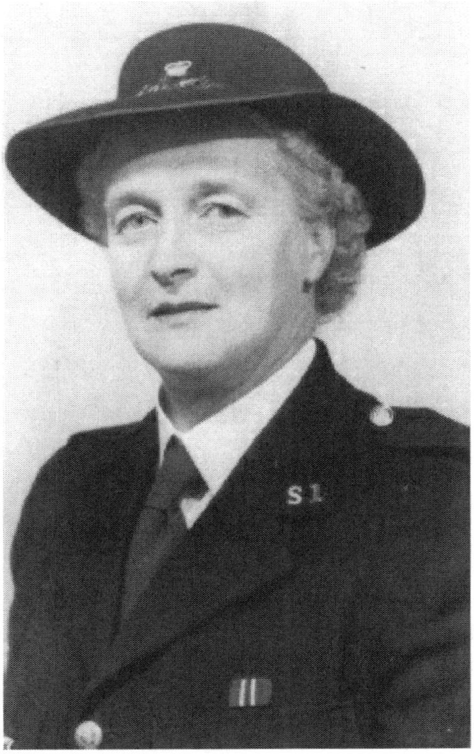

Police nurse Edna Pearce acted with care and any conditions of their internment of Japanese women and children. (Waikato Museum)

The males had been interned on Somes Island, while seven women and nine children had been moved around various locations south of Auckland and were eventually held in a dilapidated farmhouse near Pukekohe. A 37-year-old New Zealand police nurse, Edna Bertha Pearce, was placed in charge of their captivity, assisted by a translator and a retired couple who were live-in caretakers. Just 5 feet 4 inches tall, Edna had to ensure that the captives did not leave the property nor breach Police nurse Edna Pearce acted with care and any conditions of their internment. She spent the days teaching English, giving the children school lessons, procuring rice for their meals and censoring letters.

It fell to Edna Pearce to formally identify two of the women and four children who had been under her care, all victims of the crash. It was her first experience in a mortuary. Afterwards she campaigned to ensure the surviving women and children received proper medical attention. She was later recognised for her devotion in caring for the survivors, and accompanied the internees to Sydney by ship on 1 November 1943. After the war, some of her duties involved escorting royalty and celebrities and attending VIP functions, and she served the last part of her career in Hamilton, retiring in 1966. The volunteers who helped Edna Pearce with caretaking duties were recognised with an award made to their families by the police in 2006. In the same year, one of the survivors of the crash, then aged 94, also received a presentation while visiting New Zealand from Tokyo.

For many years, until being removed for motorway construction in the 1980s, the remains of the crash served as a magnet for souvenir hunters in dinghies. It is rumoured that somebody still has the navigator's map folder and someone else found a human hand. John Wisda's parents came to New Zealand in 1968, curious to visit the country where their son had miraculously survived the inferno, and were given a special tour around Whenuapai.

John Wisda was devastated in 2003 when he was informed by a television crew that there had been women and children in the compartment behind him on that fateful night, and that so many of them had perished in the crash.

17

OUR OF A BLACK SKY

The Frankton tornado 1948

Hamilton is not a city known for natural disasters. When it experienced something significant – the Frankton tornado of 1948 – it took the rest of the country a long time to appreciate the reality. It was a genuine tornado. Houses were twirled around. Others were completely splintered. Cars and other vehicles were crushed. Façades of buildings fell, often on unsuspecting locals. Window glass and roofing iron sheared through the air. Spouting was wrapped around telegraph poles. Human beings were catapulted.

These days tornadoes seem far more common than they used to be. It has been suggested that global warming and changing climate patterns have made the skies more turbulent. NIWA reports that tornado activity in New Zealand has picked up since 2000. It has also been suggested that increasing media coverage of such events has given the impression that tornadoes are more common than they really are.

After Westland in the South Island, the western side of the North Island is the most likely area for tornadoes to strike New Zealand. On average more than 30 tornadoes hit the country each year. Most of them are small and many touch down in sparsely populated areas. Consequently there are usually few victims and less damage than might be the case if New Zealand was a densely populated country.

On 6 December 2012 the following headline appeared in the New Zealand media: 'Three dead after Auckland storm and tornadoes.' It was an unusual occurrence, but a few older folk were transported back to a time and place when it was genuinely reckoned that 'this sort of thing will probably never happen again.'

The time was 1948 and the place was Hamilton. On 25 August of that year, a tornado descended. In a country known for its usually benign climate the tornado came out of the blue, or more precisely, the black. It wasn't the sort of weather event New Zealanders of the 1940s expected to see. Certainly not in Hamilton, a town where even then aspersions were cast about the fact that very little ever seemed to happen in the inland Waikato town. In a newspaper editorial after the tornado, it was reported that there was no area less subject to violent winds in New Zealand.

Today, few people know anything about the Hamilton tornado of 1948 or even that it occurred. Awareness of the Auckland tornado and recent 'weather bombs' on the West Coast are more familiar reminders of the vagaries of New Zealand weather. The 1948 Hamilton tornado killed three people, injured 80 and destroyed or badly damaged 150 houses. When you see photos of the devastation it seems miraculous that only three people lost their lives, although many more suffered injuries ranging from minor to grievous.

A man who had been working at a garage in Kent Street, Frankton was found pinned down by heavy doors. He later died in hospital. A woman living in a Lake Road house that was lifted bodily from its section and flung across the North Island Main Trunk railway line, was found with a severe head injury from which she died. The third fatality also occurred in Lake Road. A bach was completely flattened by the twister and the body of a woman was eventually found beneath the debris.

As the tornado tore through Frankton, telephone and power poles were snapped off and many trees uprooted. In ten minutes the tornado cut a swathe over 100 metres wide. Flying roofing iron was a particular hazard and people scurried around to find protection from the missiles. There were some amazing escape stories. One house was lifted up in its entirety, twirled around like a child's toy and dumped on the opposite side of the street. Somehow the three occupants survived. Some streets suffered more than others. Every home on the Frankton Railway Station side of Keddell Street was totally destroyed.

Inten minutes the tornado cut a swathe over 100 metres wide.

Initially the people of Frankton were fascinated by the looming black cloud which appeared to touch down in the suburb of Maeroa to the north-west. A woman and her children attempted to leave their home to take a closer look at the strange phenomenon. Before they had a chance to get beyond the front hall, the house seemed to buckle in on itself and the woman and her children were thrown to the floor. The house had been sucked off its foundations and tossed around. The kitchen, bathroom and bedroom were scythed off, the roof taken away. Miraculously the only portion of the roof that remained intact was that covering the front hall where the woman and her children were bowled over. As a result they survived.

In other houses windows blew in, creating a hazard for those inside. By now some residents had been irresistibly drawn outside by the incredible roar of the tornado. Flying wreckage made this zone even more treacherous. Telegraph poles were ripped out of the ground. Miles of electric light and telephone wires were plucked up and spirited away by the tornado, never to be seen again. Even heavy objects like cars, trucks and vans were tossed into heaps of virtually unrecognisable junk.

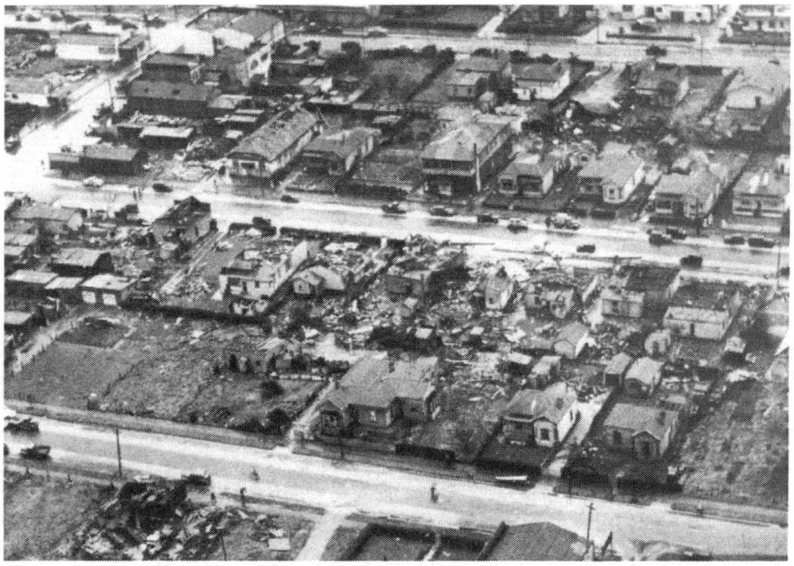

Frankton flattened. The randomness of the tornado is apparent, missing some houses but obliterating others, (Alexander Turnbull Library, 54247 1/2)

The main business area of Frankton was badly hit. The Maoriland Company's timber mill in Kent Street lost a machine shop and suffered serious damage to plant and machinery. The grocery store belonging to Mr A. Murdoch, located on the corner of Kent Street and Norton Road, was believed to be the first business struck by the tornado. Onlookers saw its veranda fly away and the walls cave in. A dairy cattle sale at the Frankton sale yards was in progress when the tornado touched down. Although fences were flattened, there was no stampede. Not by the cattle anyway.

Telegraph poles were ripped out of the ground.

At the time it was considered by some badly rattled Hamilton citizens that the tornado had touched down on the northern outskirts of the city. Others claimed it had hit the suburb of Maeroa, or perhaps Forest Lake. Others were adamant that the tornado simply dropped out of the sky in the heart of Frankton, although it was significant at this stage that these same people were aware of a mass of what looked like paper swirling within the tornado clouds. The mass was in fact sheets of lethal roofing iron, suggesting that the tornado had already wreaked havoc to the north of Frankton.

Having cut a swathe through the business area of Frankton, the tornado continued on its terrifying course through several nearby residential streets, then disappeared over Tower Hill into Hamilton West. Here it passed between Hamilton Lake and the main thoroughfare of Victoria Street, damaging roofs in Anglesea and Collingwood Streets before crossing the Waikato River, where it caused further damage in Wellington, Naylor and Grey Streets in Hamilton East. Its final calling card was minor damage at Hillcrest High School on the outskirts, before passing into open country towards Tamahere. Debris from the tornado was cast over the plains as far as Bruntwood and Hautapu near the town of Cambridge.

Once the tornado had passed, scenes of devastation lay all around. After the initial shock, rescue operations were set in motion. Virtually every policeman in Hamilton was mobilised to assess and assist. All police stations in the Waikato area were alerted and extra police resources were rushed to the scene. A group of policemen were even dispatched south from Auckland.

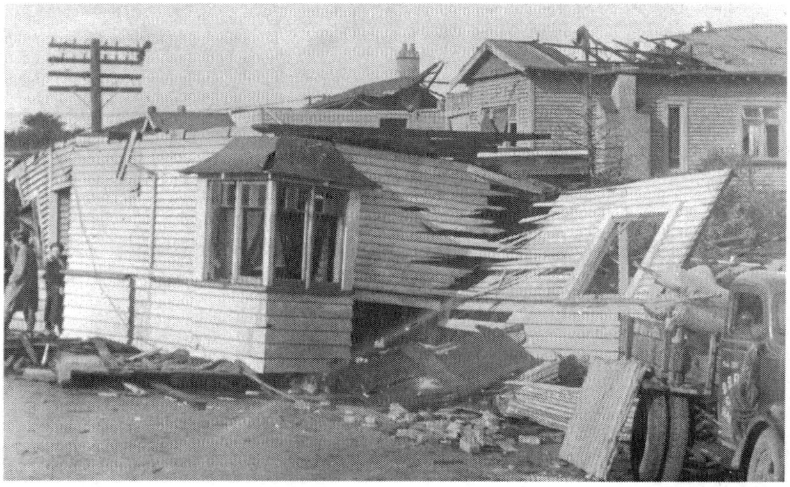

Ordinary families faced unimaginable damage to their houses. (Hamilton City Libraries, HCL-2631)

Of course medical professionals were assisting casualties almost before the tornado had died out. Ambulances and private vehicles rushed the injured to hospital. In keeping with the generous and homogeneous nature of New Zealand society at the time, hundreds of Hamilton residents offered temporary accommodation to those who had lost their homes. Some houses were salvageable, but in the meantime it was deemed too dangerous for their owners to return to them. For those who could not be accommodated in this manner, several local halls were converted into temporary hotels for the homeless.

One of the saving graces of the tornado was the fact that leaking gas did not prove a problem. Fires fuelled by gas could have been catastrophic. It had been a priority at the outset of the rescue for the gas supply to be cut off and broken pipes to be repaired. Amazingly the electric power was back up and running in areas of Frankton by six o'clock the same evening. Some of the more seriously affected parts were without power for several days.

Another remarkable feature of the tornado was that, although many residents had fires burning in open fireplaces, no serious blaze started in the wreckage as the wind hurled burning embers around. Obviously the heavy torrential rain that continued to fall during the tornado dampened things down. A further hazard presented itself when live power lines crackled on wet pavements until the power was cut off.

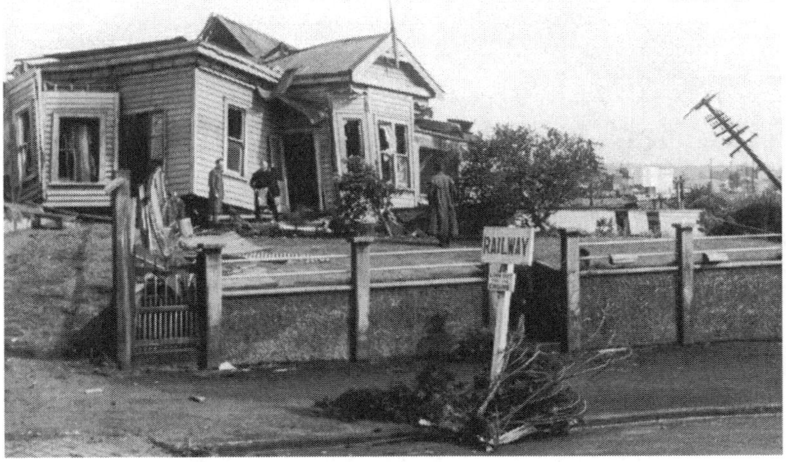

Badly bent out of shape. One of the three fatalities occurred in this house, (Hamilton City Libraries, HCL-09892)

Amidst all the grimness there were occasional flashes of humour. Not long after the tornado had passed, a woman was seen at the top of a ladder trying to retrieve her washing that had been whipped away to lodge in one of the trees that hadn't been snapped off or uprooted.

In a wasteland that reminded some of scenes from the London blitz of World War Two, it seemed a miracle that only three people died. A figure of closer to 300 struck some people as being more likely, given the amount of damage. While the experience of those who lived through the tornado was undoubtedly horrifying, the carnage could have been so much worse.

There was an uncanny silence just before the tornado and in the moments after it had passed. It was accompanied by heavy rain that fell almost horizontally, yet was blown skyward just as it was about to touch the ground. A roaring noise, like a thousand goods trains, assailed and disoriented. Lightning flashed, thunder boomed. Adults felt as if they'd descended into hell as their lives and livelihoods changed before their very eyes. Parents were especially concerned about the terror being meted out to petrified children.

Fortunately it only lasted ten minutes but most survivors were badly shocked. After the tornado they wandered around aimlessly, some collecting what possessions they could, others unable to grasp the enormity of what had just happened. The police were assisted by Air Force officers from the Te Rapa base and Army personnel from Hopuhopu as the disaster scene was evaluated. Such officers would provide support if looting became a problem. Tarpaulins were spread everywhere over the stricken areas, for the torrential rain continued into the next day.

Curious onlookers, either on foot or in cars, hindered rescue and clean-up operations and local rubberneckers were advised to keep clear. The damage to houses was severe. An early estimate identified 78 badly damaged houses, 57 less badly damaged and 38 slightly damaged. These figures were later formalised and the initial total of 173 damaged houses became 150. Amazement was again expressed that amidst such destruction the death toll was so low.

Soon plans were being made for rebuilding. At the time there was a labour shortage, but the problem was alleviated by deploying Returned Services trade trainees. Fletcher Construction from Auckland also supplied much in the way of materials, and other firms and organisations were generous in helping to get Frankton back on its feet. It had been New Zealand's most lethal tornado, yet it only lasted ten minutes. The damage it caused seemed to be the work of a far more prolonged weather event. Yet despite the amount of damage, a year or two later it was remarked how quickly the suburb of Frankton was repaired and rebuilt. The government of the day, led by Prime Minister Peter Fraser, provided impetus by pushing for the rebuilding programme to be given high priority. Fraser and several other prominent politicians visited the site; according to the *Waikato Times,* the ruination had a profound effect on them.

In 2004 New Zealand was reminded of the lethal properties of tornadoes when one struck near Waitara, Taranaki. Again three people lost their lives and severe property damage occurred. In 2007 a swarm of at least 12 tornadoes landed near the Taranaki coast. Oakura, south-west of New Plymouth, ended up with more than 50 houses suffering serious damage, due to two tornadoes hitting the town.

Today, the Frankton tornado seems slightly unreal. But the disaster was not an abstract event. Real people were affected. This was confirmed when, in the pages of the *Waikato Times* the day after the tragedy, three death notices recorded the family and funeral details of the three who died. Each notice included the following: 'On August 25, 1948, result of tornado.'

18

A ROGUE WAVE

The sinking of the *Ranui* 1950

In 1950 Mount Maunganui was already one of New Zealand's most popular holiday destinations. In egalitarian days when bach ownership was within the financial capabilities of many, hundreds of baches sat on the headland, either looking out over the excellent surf beach or fronting the placid Tauranga Harbour. Larger, more elaborate beach houses were springing up too, for in 1950 the New Zealand economy was burgeoning. It was five years after the end of World War Two and New Zealand, like other British allies, was receiving the spoils of war. Britain bought as much of our agricultural produce as we could provide and Kiwis began to grow fat. The 'golden years' of the 1950s began to glow. Mount Maunganui, at this time, was a favourite holiday Mecca for farmers from the Waikato, who prospered as Britain bought more of our meat and dairy produce, and the shop-keepers and merchants who gloried in the flowdown from the farmers. There was no trickledown in those days. The benefits were more immediate and direct.

The mood of people was positive. To be on holiday in Tauranga and Mount Maunganui in 1950 was to have made it, at least in the North Island. There was a certain status attached to holidaying at Tauranga and 'The Mount', particularly for young adults. It was where 'the action' was. The prettiest girls and the 'tall, dark and handsome' young men gathered at the Bay of Plenty resort to preen and be seen. Some even ventured into the water, occasionally on the harbour side of the isthmus, but more likely in the even breakers crashing onto the fashionable white sands of Mount Maunganui Beach.

Against this background, summer could sometimes lose its golden sheen. Three days after Christmas, 28 December was not a day graced by clear blue skies, pure white sands and fetching brown bodies. It was stormy, and heavy downpours had turned the white sand to a muddy brown. The brown bodies donned clothing that hid the tans but defied the stinging wind.

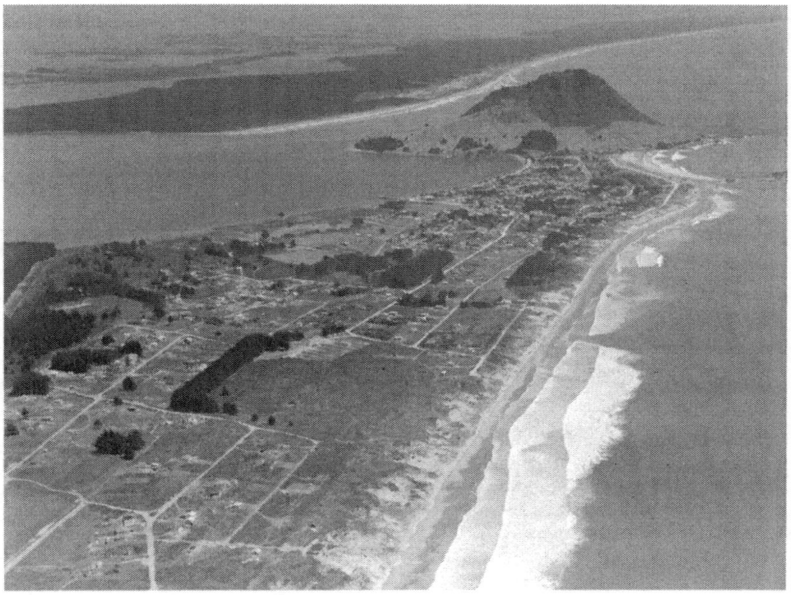

Mount Maunganui in 1950. The Ranui came to grief at the mouth of the harbour. (Alexander Turnbull Library, Whites Aviation Photographs, Ref: WA-23773-F)

Kiwis can be less than cautious during their summer holidays. Just because the sun disappears and the ocean churns up into pale green waves as big as a house, you don't have to slink into the great indoors – be it tent, caravan or bach – and wait out the mean, unseasonal weather. No, these were the Christmas holidays, your basic Kiwi 'two-weeker', when hardworking New Zealanders deserved the best weather, and if something different turned up you didn't have to keep your boat under wraps just because the sea got a bit rough.

However, our history as amateur mariners is peppered with nautical risk-taking. This might be Godzone, but a merciful God didn't always get involved when the foolhardy pitted themselves against unfavourable seas in boats that were puny at best. Then there was the simple reality of Kiwis having generous access to the ocean. We tended to believe that the ocean, in all its moods, belonged to us and we had a right to expect good behaviour whenever we went down to the sea in boats. The reality was less childlike.

Launches sink and even large fishing boats can. Certainly dinghies and runabouts come to grief in New Zealand's teeming waters. It's the negative price we pay for inhabiting an island nation where most live within a short distance of the sea. The more hard-nosed of us expect to read about people in boats coming to grief occasionally. We expect drownings in such situations from time to time – particularly in summer.

The day a passenger launch capsized while negotiating the entrance to Tauranga Harbour it was summer: 28 December 1950. However, it was a wild sort of day weatherwise. No one expected that and no one thought the boat would flip over either. It was virtually within the safe confines of the harbour. Certainly no one expected 22 of the 23 people on board to lose their lives.

Certainly no one expected 22 of the 23 people on board to lose their lives.

After the era of the great New Zealand shipwrecks when large, oceangoing vessels foundered and often hundreds died on or near our coastline, the numbers who drowned in boating accidents reduced considerably. Admittedly the sea still claimed many New Zealanders, but not in mass disasters and the number of deaths in most boating accidents was rarely into double figures.

This is the reason that the wreck of the *Ranui* at the confluence of Tauranga Harbour created such a shock. In 1950 it was virtually unheard of to lose 22 people in a single incident. New Zealanders could imagine a situation in which 22 lives were lost miles out to sea, even on a wild, desolate rock-strewn shore miles from anywhere. But the *Ranui* was only a mile off Mount Maunganui when the boat's captain radioed his position to the marine radio station at Tauranga. At around 6p.m. the boat was only 200 metres offshore, already inside the harbour bar, when all hell broke loose.

The *Ranui* was described as a 'stout little craft'. It was 45 feet long and 14 feet wide. It was a 'working' boat with a licence to carry 72 people. It was often chartered by fishing parties, particularly those who wanted to try their hand at big-game fishing in the waters around Mayor Island, roughly 25 miles off the coast.

The fact that the *Ranui* was built of kauri, a much-sought-after New Zealand hardwood, lent the vessel an air of impregnability. Moreover, she had entered service only a few weeks before she was chartered to take fishermen and campers to Mayor Island on 28 December 1950.

Her emergency equipment was impressive too. She had three watertight bulkheads in a vessel that did not, compulsorily, require such measures. Her five life-rafts were each capable of accommodating 16 passengers. As back-up, the *Ranui* also carried four lifebuoys and twelve life jackets.

The *Ranui* left Tauranga around 8a.m. with a crew of three and over 20 passengers. Although the seas were rough at the outset, the overriding, cavalier approach of 'she'll be right' – or 'she'll come right' – comforted those who felt initially uneasy. The *Ranui* would be at sea for most of the day and the weather and high seas would eventually settle down.

Rough trips were not unknown and the *Ranui* confronted one. Yet it was portentous that the skipper Geoffrey Harnett, ten minutes into the journey, considered turning back to Tauranga port. The Christmas holidays are probably the hardest time to make hard decisions. Everyone succumbs to the celebratory mood and reason can fly out the window. Harnett had made promises to transport campers to Mayor Island and he didn't want to break a promise. The *Ranui* forged onward.

The fact that nearly everyone on board was violently seasick as the doughty launch was tossed around by the broken seas didn't seem to sound warning bells. In fact, several choruses of popular songs were struck up as passengers attempted to take their minds off the worsening situation. 'I've got a lovely bunch of coconuts' was a favourite. Others sought safety and reassurance in the *Ranui's* wheelhouse. Five or six passengers left the launch at Mayor Island. They were the lucky ones. Not so fortunate were the young couple who climbed on board the *Ranui* after a holiday on the island.

Eventually, after fighting her way through the open ocean, the *Ranui* approached the Tauranga Harbour entrance. The worst of the trip seemed to be over. 'I've got a lovely bunch of coconuts' came wafting in on the inshore wind from time to time, but mostly it was the roar of the sea and the crashing of the surf that predominated. Then, out of the blue, the predatory sea struck.

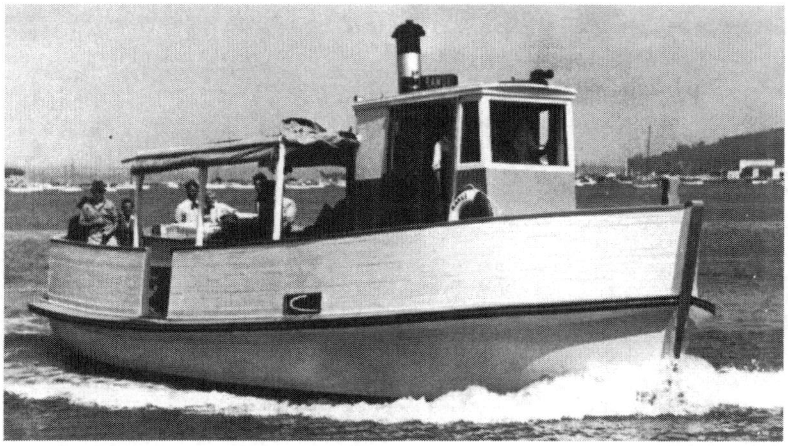

The Ranui in happier times. [Bay of Plenty Times and Tauranga City Libraries)

The accident, the overturning of the *Ranui,* appeared to be a freak of nature – the sort of backhander Mother Nature seldom dealt to Kiwis. Admittedly the *Ranui* had some challenging waves to negotiate as she sought to enter the harbour. A series of waves larger than earlier ones crashed down on the starboard side and then a rogue wave came up under her stern. The *Ranui* was catapulted clear of the water and in a second was nose-diving downwards on the front of the wave. She then flipped over, casting people in all directions. The capsize appeared to be the work of a single wave.

It was a moment of aberration. The *Ranui* had appeared to be making steady progress in admittedly rough seas. But the wave that did the damage was unlike any that had been seen before. It arrived suddenly – and lethally.

If there had been cause for concern amongst the people on the *Ranui* you would have imagined that life jackets would already have been donned, but when the wave struck it appeared that people had no time to take protective action. The rogue wave swept the life-rafts beyond reach. People were dragged overboard or trapped in the wheelhouse, where several had sought safety as the sea cut up.

With the benefit of hindsight and being aware of New Zealanders' often cavalier approach to water safety, observers later questioned the lack of awareness of the trouble the *Ranui* was in. A huge dollop of Kiwi complacency was obvious. Very few if any boats of *Ranui*'s size had come to grief in similar circumstances. Besides, it was the Christmas holidays in Godzone, where life was good now that the war was over. Why, the jovial passengers had been singing their hearts out as the *Ranui* cut through the waves. Whether the singing was generated to disguise the anxieties of often novice sailors was a point of discussion in the days following the disaster.

The attempt by the *Ranui* to negotiate the heads had been witnessed by many. At that time of day, most locals and holidaymakers would have done for the day and many were strolling along the beach, defying the elements, or perusing the ocean from lounge windows. Some had even tried the sporting breakers of the ocean beach. In between dips, toasts would have been drunk to the best country in the world in which to raise children. A country like no other, where Jack was as good as his master, and both were welcome to take their holidays overlooking the golden sands and even waves of Mount Maunganui, with a quart bottle of beer not too far away.

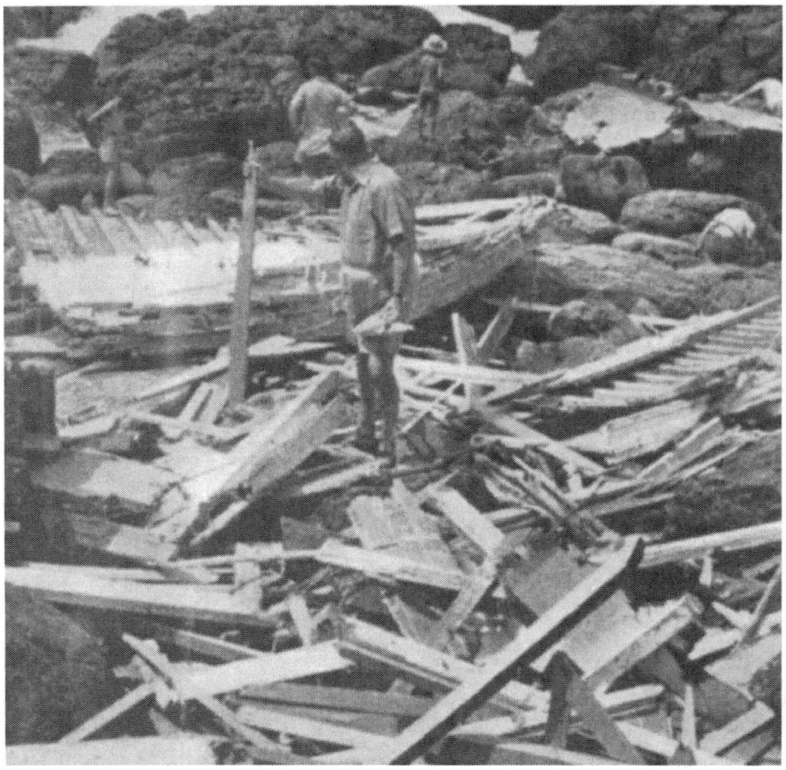

The Ranui in ruins on the rocks (also opposite). (Alexander Turnbull Library, New Zealand Shipping News, Ref: IRN 1662377 PA Coll 0785 1 096)

It seemed significant that one of the first eye-witnesses of the *Ranui's* plight hightailed it to the Oceanside Hotel. He had to run half a mile, but such was the horror of seeing the boat upended and all those people being cast about like rag dolls, it was more of a sprint. The alarm was sounded from the Oceanside Hotel as happy imbibers turned ashen at the news. Members of the Mount Maunganui Surf Life Saving Club were soon on the scene. If ever lives needed saving it was now. Even in the time it had taken the sprinting eye-witness to seek help, most of the lives had probably been lost.

You had to admire the efforts of the rescuers. Many of the bodies were dashed ashore on the jagged rocks that studded the coastline around the base of Mount Maunganui. The rescuers themselves were in danger as they sought to bring them ashore in the high seas. Several were badly injured as the cruel sea cast them onto the same rocks that showed no respect to the victims of the *Ranui.* Two rescuers were admitted to Tauranga Hospital, such was the gravity of their injuries, while others were stretchered off in states of exhaustion to hotel beds, where no doubt a fortifying quart or two of lager eased the pain.

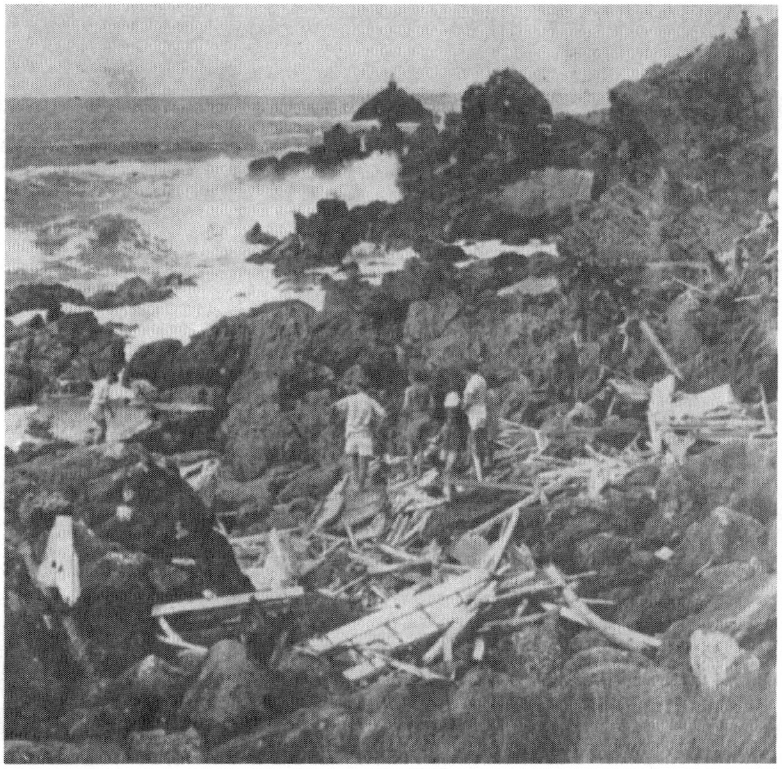

Someone said that the formerly jovial locals and high-spirited holiday-makers who were involved in that brave but battering rescue attempt showed something of the wartime spirit. By now the ocean was so savage that the good ship *Ranui* was splintered. Only pieces of wood less than six feet in length remained, to be washed ashore as sad remnants of an extraordinary event. Half a beer crate bobbed on the foamy breakers.

By the following day thirteen bodies had been recovered. The high seas continued for the next few days and a week passed before the rest of the bodies came ashore. The loss of so many lives was traumatic. Most people knew someone on board. Tauranga was a town of only 7000 people in those days.

Phillip Smith, a 19-year-old deckhand on the *Ranui,* was the only survivor – and he only just made it. He had been in the wheelhouse when the boat capsized and twice he snagged his leg on the wheel. In the end he twisted his ankle while wrenching his leg clear. Once he was in the ocean, the *Ranui* still posed a threat. He suffered several knocks to the head as he collided with the boat. He could have been rendered unconscious. Then there was the business of getting to shore and safety. The undertow dragged him under, but finally a massive wave caught hold of him and cast him over the more dangerous rocks. A smaller wave might have dumped him on top of them, a fatal outcome for several passengers. As it was, Smith ended up clinging to a rock close to shore, from where three lifesavers dragged him to safety. *Smith ended up clinging to a rock close to shore.*

Only one survivor. The holiday spirit died. Many holidaymakers left for home early. The sinking of the *Ranui* cast a pall of gloom over Mount Maunganui and Tauranga for a long time. The sense of bonhomie and 'she'll be right' was temporarily buried as everyone tried to come to terms with the tragedy. Many boaties were reluctant to put to sea, certainly to cross over the harbour bar into the open ocean. Internally, many carried with them a feeling of depression and deep sympathy for those who had lost their lives, and the families and friends of the victims. 'So much for the war being over,' some said. It didn't feel like a homecoming parade when 22 innocent people could be accounted for by a rogue wave. Would it have felt better somehow if it had been a torpedo or a Jap mine that caused the sinking? To think that good old Mother Nature could throw you a curve ball when you were feeling about as good as you could. And just when things were getting back to normal after the war.

19

HOLLOW VICTORY

Wellington to Lyttelton yachting tragedy 1951

In 1940 a yacht race was held to commemorate Wellington's centenary. The racing between Lyttelton Harbour and Port Nicholson was strenuous and the competition keen. It was a popular event, so when it was Canterbury's turn to celebrate its centenary in 1951, it made perfect sense to stage a race going in the opposite direction.

Back in 1951, yacht races were not the high-profile extravaganzas that would later characterise the America's Cup contests. In fact, yacht racing was a minority sporting activity. It was always a bit elitist because of the cost factor, even in a country where egalitarianism was a prime cornerstone of society.

It was OK to muck about in boats. In fact, many Kiwis owned or had access to basic runabouts and modest launches, which were propelled by outboard motors. Yachts and sails seemed to belong to a different kind of New Zealander. This was never more aptly demonstrated than when Ron Jarden, the champion All Black wing of the early 1950s, retired early and was next sighted, in the sporting arena, representing his country in the Admiral's Cup international yachting series in Britain. Ron Jarden had been a champion of the majority in rugby-besotted New Zealand. As a yachtsman he was obviously just as skilled. It was just that yachting was a bit more than messing around in boats – perhaps a bit exclusive. And Jarden was a stockbroker in days when the stock market was not yet the temple of 1980s yuppies.

What made the 1951 centennial yacht race between Wellington and Lyttelton typically Kiwi – something we could all identify with – was the risk factor involved. Several serious disasters occurred in New Zealand in the early 1950s, at a time when Kiwis in general were prepared to chance their arms in the buoyant, sometimes over-confident post-war years. Now that they'd help beat Germany and Japan, nothing could get in their way – not even the threat of unfavourable weather.

Twenty yachts set out from Clyde Quay Wharf on 23 January 1951, bound for Lyttelton. It was estimated that the 180-mile race would take between 1½ and 5 days to complete, with 36 hours being a common expectation. There were high levels of excitement as the flotilla entered Cook Strait. One of the favourites to win the race, *Restless,* was forced to pull out early when it lost its mast. Three other boats suffered minor damage and were also forced to turn back. The remaining yachts crossed Cook Strait in reasonable shape. The weather was described as fair, with an easterly wind blowing. To all intents and purposes it was full steam ahead for Lyttelton.

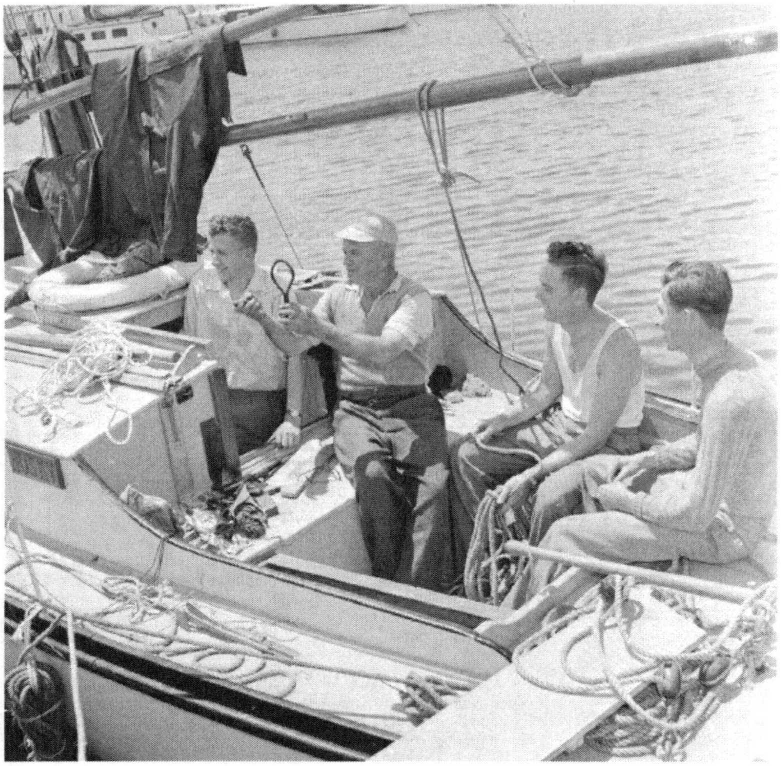

A relaxed crew prepares for the Wellington to Lyttelton yacht race. (Alexander Turnbull Library, Ref: 114/252/05-F)

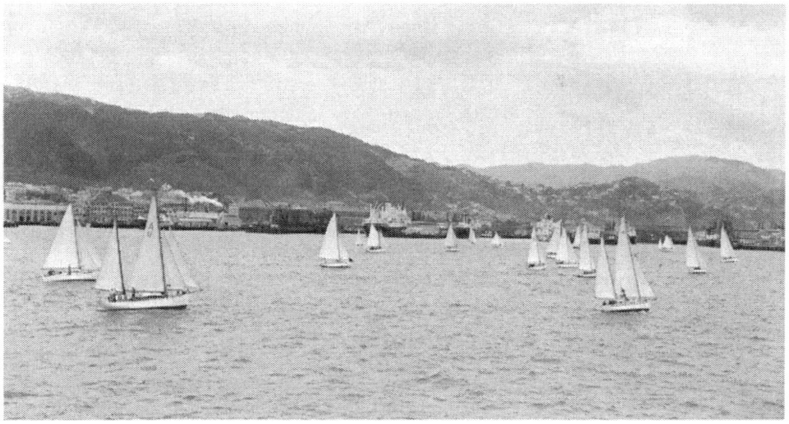

The yachts sail out of Wellington Harbour at the start of the race. All seemed in order at this stage. (Alexander Turnbull Library, Ref: 114/255/06-G)

All contestants should have been concerned, though, when George Brasell, an experienced seaman and skipper of a yacht called *Joy,* withdrew from the race. Brasell was unable to put his finger on any specific reason for *Joy*'s withdrawal, other than to mention that something seemed wrong and his boat and crew pulled out of it before whatever it was arrived.

Obviously it was the weather, and although the race began in conditions that were described by some as fair, it was significant that others described the weather conditions as dodgy, and – more significantly – growing worse by the hour. But 'the boats must go through' was the prevailing attitude of many participants and officials. Not George Brasell's though.

That evening the wind turned southerly, indicating the formation of a storm front. By the following evening a severe storm had developed with gale-force winds and turbulent seas. George Brasell, a Wellingtonian, was only too aware of the sudden development of storms in the waters around Cook Strait. Six yachts pulled out of the race on 24 January. Either that or they were disqualified for using their engines to combat the turbulent seas. Many returned to Wellington where they found shelter along the coast. Others remained at sea in their attempts to ride out the storm.

From this point the centennial yacht race became an exercise in survival on the open ocean. It wasn't until the morning of the 26th that *Astral,* a yacht that hadn't been heard from since the storm descended, was spotted from the air. A fishing trawler named *Tawera* put to sea to assist the yacht, which had lost its mast in the storm. A tow-line was made fast between the *Tawera* and the *Astral,* but when this was severed the *Tawera* hovered near the yacht throughout the stormy night. The following morning it was decided to abandon the *Astral.* The crew jumped overboard and were picked up by the *Tawera* some distance from Lyttelton, near the mouth of the Clarence River.

The following morning it was decided to abandon the Astral.

The rescue trawler *Tawera* was skippered by George Brasell, the skipper who had had the foresight to turn back early in the centennial race. In an unusual twist, he was now active in the rescue of the *Astral*'s crew.

Such was the gallantry, seamanship and endurance displayed by Brasell and his crew that they were later honoured by the Royal Humane Society.

Several other yachts were reported missing and the situation was becoming dire. Then there was good news and bad. Two yachts that were among the missing reported in on 27 and 28 January. However, two more, the *Aurora* and *Argo,* were still missing. Then came a pivotal point in the search. The yacht *Husky* was found near Owhiro Bay, Wellington, but its four crew members were missing, presumed drowned. Those who had been on board were the skipper, Arthur Clements of Lyttelton, Kevin Clark also of Lyttelton, and two Christchurch yachtsmen, Kelvin Hopkinson and Harvey Mason.

On 29 January, *Aurora* was able to make communication with an overseas freighter heading for Lyttelton. That left just *Argo* unaccounted for, and hopes were not high for the boat or its six crew members, all Wellingtonians. They were John Young, the skipper, Clarence Pickering, Malcolm Mace, Allan Henderson, Alan Baker and Robert Fielding.

The official search for the *Argo* was cancelled on the evening of 29 January. The authorities in charge of the search claimed they had covered the area where the yacht was likely to be. An agreement was reached that the search would be reconvened if evidence of the yacht's location emerged.

Despite the looming tragedy, the centennial race continued. The possible loss of ten yachtsmen and other uncertainties did not lead to the official cancellation of the race. In fact, the sloop *Tawhiri* of Nelson was declared the winner – and indeed the only boat to finish the race – when it entered Lyttelton Harbour and approached the finish line in 'spectacular fashion', according to newspapers around the country. It was a somewhat hollow victory. Other yachts made it to Lyttelton – the *Caplin, Fantasy, Galatea* and *Windswift* – but they were disqualified for using their engines during the race.

Aurora, once its location had been confirmed, announced that it hoped to find its way to Lyttelton to claim second place when it heard of *Tawhiri's* triumph. Once again there seemed to be little concern for the lost boats and men, just a single-minded desire to make something of the race. The crew of *Aurora* should have lowered their expectations, for like many others, they were disqualified for using their yacht's engines during the storm. They were eventually over the time limit as well.

Although *Aurora* reported to the foreign freighter that it was heading for Lyttelton, it had earlier been trying to land at Napier, miles to the north, to reassure family and friends, when it broke the seal on its engine. This was when disqualification became inevitable. After the storm the would-be second-placed yacht resumed its journey, finally pulling into Kaikoura on 1 February after running low on food.

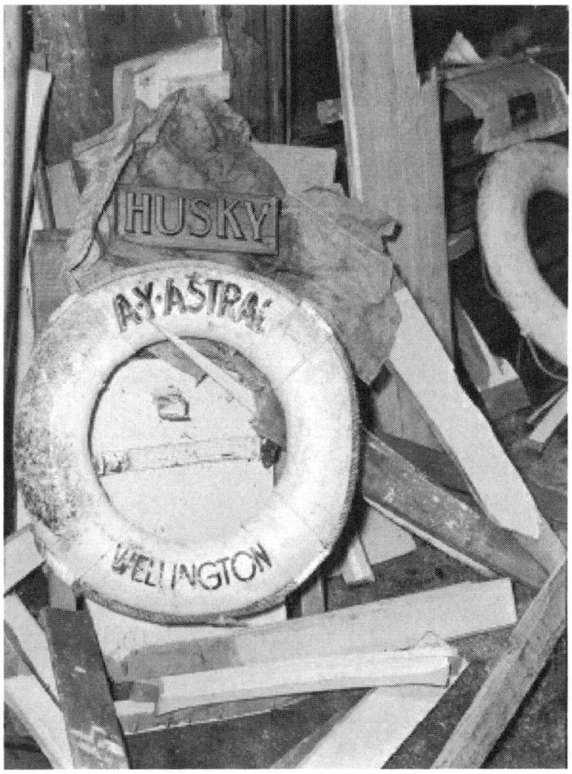

Wreckage from the ill-fated Husky and the more fortunate Astral.
(Alexander Turnbull Library, Ref: 114/257/01-G)

So *Tawhiri* 'won' the Wellington to Lyttelton yacht race. No one came second. Nor third. It had also won the race held to celebrate Wellington's centenary in 1940. The wreck of the *Husky* had already been found and its crew declared dead. Some other competitors like the *Astral* and *Aurora* and those who had turned back to seek shelter in Wellington or around the fringes of the harbour, could be accounted for. But not the *Argo.* The search resumed in early February when weak radio signals from the yacht were picked up near East Cape, a long way to the north. Then a lifebuoy and cushion believed to belong to the lost yacht were washed up at Palliser Bay, Wellington. It's a long way from Palliser Bay to East Cape.

The air and sea search for the *Argo* continued. The RNZAF and other aviation operators eventually covered 165,000 square nautical miles (566,000 square kilometres) but there was no sign of the missing yacht. Friends and family of the missing crew conducted private searches, but these too were fruitless. On 12 February the Minister of Defence, T. L. MacDonald announced that the search had been called off.

Later that year a magisterial enquiry was held into the loss of the *Husky* and *Argo.* It was revealed that the *Argo* had collided with *Nanette,* another competitor, early in the race. As a result *Argo* lost its bobstay, a rope used to hold down the bowsprit and aid stability. This made the boat less seaworthy and may have contributed to its demise. The enquiry also made recommendations regarding the running of future yacht races, with a greater emphasis on safety.

The race became one of New Zealand's most bizarre disasters. It was bad enough that looming deteriorating weather was disregarded. It was almost as if wartime motivation was still at play, although the war had finished over five years earlier. Perhaps the sanctity of human life was still played down, as if wartime conditions still prevailed. Or was it just that Kiwis underestimated the sea and overestimated their maritime skills? And then there was the extraordinary running of the race, long after the storm developed and the threat of heavy loss of life was bearing down on officials and surviving competitors. The race was not called off. Ten men, in all likelihood more, were probably dead, yet still the *Tawhiri* was welcomed across the finishing line. The Nelson Harbour Board sent a letter of praise to the 'successful' crew and authorised the harbourmaster to meet the *Tawhiri* on her triumphant return to Nelson some weeks later. Meanwhile searches were continuing for lost yachts and for those who would never come home.

The loss of ten lives made the Wellington to Lyttelton centennial race the worst calamity in the yachting history of New Zealand and the greatest disaster in New Zealand sport.

20

BECAUSE IT WAS THERE

The Mount Egmont climbing accident 1953

Taranaki folk are proud of their mountain, Mount Taranaki (as it is more commonly known today). They were proud of it back in 1953 too, when it was generally referred to as Mt Egmont. It rose 8260 feet above the plains and was remarkable for being an almost perfect cone. The fact that it was a stand-alone physical phenomenon added to its allure. It was as if Mother Nature, as an afterthought, or because she had one perfect cone left over, needed somewhere to plonk a mountain and noting that the Taranaki plains were largely unencumbered as they sloped down to the sea, decided on its resting place.

Mt Egmont was too perfect a mountain not to attract the attention of those who would wish to climb her. Her near-perfect lines were irresistible to experienced mountain climbers but also attracted the attention of awestruck amateurs. 'Because it was there' is often cited as a good enough reason for human beings to want to pit themselves against a mountain – to climb the devil and be able to say you had conquered its scope and majesty. You didn't have to be a supreme athlete to have a go. You just needed to be committed, keen – and careful. Half the people of Taranaki province had either climbed the mountain, or trudged its lower slopes, or dreamed of one day making it to the top.

On 26 July 1953, it was the turn of a group of nurses to have a go. July 1953: the middle of a New Zealand winter. It was an extraordinary year for New Zealand and New Zealanders. Edmund Hillary climbed Everest, the first man to do so. The fact that a little-known bee-keeper from Pukekohe could become the first human being to conquer the world's highest mountain led to feelings back home that a lot of us had mountaineering blood in our veins. Hillary's extraordinary achievement in the Himalayas certainly had many New Zealanders looking at our mountains in a different light. Was some of the motivation of the nurses who set out to conquer Egmont in July fired by Edmund Hillary's achievements?

And then there was the looming prospect of the newly crowned Queen Elizabeth visiting New Zealand at the end of the year. But if Kiwis had been able to look into a crystal ball, they would have seen a murky event that rather put the dampener on 1953: the Tangiwai rail disaster on Christmas Eve. It was a year of highs and lows.

On 26 July, the nurses headed out on a nice enough winter's day to climb Mt Egmont. A few male climbers were also in the party, including Keith Russell, the Taranaki Alpine Club's chief guide. He was one of the club's most experienced climbers and added a level of assurance as the excited nurses began their ascent from the Tahurangi Hut at 11a.m. The late departure would prove to be significant later.

In all there were 31 climbers, divided into six separate ropes, each attached to a number of climbers. Three were led by men and three by women – Beryl Robinson, L. Eades and A. Vickers. Because of his experience, Keith Russell had seven climbers on his rope, while the others supported four or five. Keith Russell was something of a mountaineering legend in Taranaki, having climbed the Alps in Europe and once ascended the Matterhorn without a guide.

By 3.45p.m. all climbers had made it to the summit.

By 3.45p.m. all climbers had made it to the summit. The ascent hadn't been easy. Icy conditions prevailed and a strong, piercing wind blew. The wind cast snow back into the steps they cut as they climbed. Ideally the steps would have been available for the descent, particularly as the light was dimming rapidly at that time of year. However, it was necessary for another climber, Derek Quickfall, who was wearing crampons and not part of the larger party, to lead the descent and chip out new steps. This process took up valuable time while the light was closing in fast.

Keith Russell's group headed down first. At the Tahurangi Hut, concern was expressed at the late arrival of the party. The Alpine Club's captain, Tom Herbert, felt reassured when he was able to monitor them through binoculars, climbing down into Snow Valley. Herbert knew that once the sun set, softened snow froze over and became very slippery. And yet the path Keith Russell's group was taking – the snow face above Hongi's Bluff – was part of the usual route for those ascending or descending via Snow Valley.

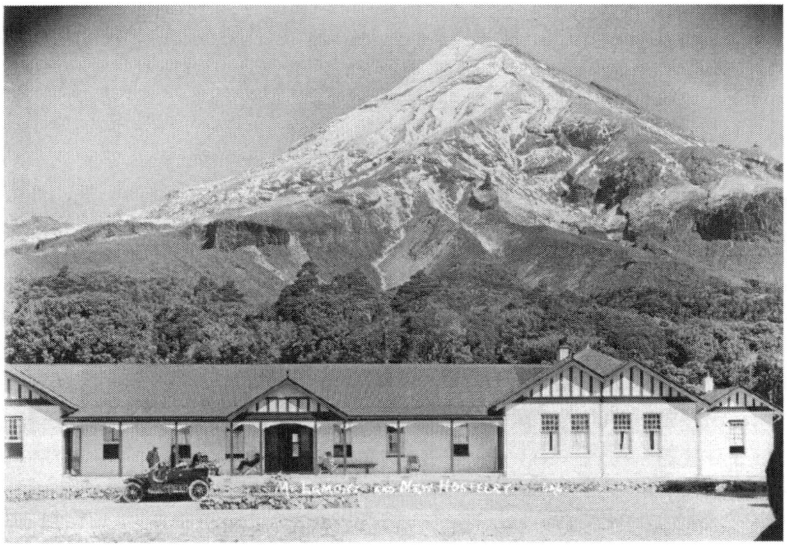

The mountain looms over North Egmont Hostel. The victims were moved here from the Nissen Hut. (Alexander Turnbull Library, Ref: 1/2-001 273-G)

As a precaution, however, Herbert had dispatched Derek Quickfall, Ron Shorter and Barry Hartley, Taranaki Alpine Club members, back up the mountain to help. Conditions were now freezing and a vicious wind pounded the climbers as the sky got darker. One rope group of four slipped and slid 200 yards before

Dick Williams, a 20-year-old member of the Taranaki Alpine Club, threw himself in the group's path, stopped its plunge and probably saved four lives.

Then at 6.30p.m., as Keith Russell's party was crossing the slope, one of the nurses dropped her ski stick. Russell moved to assist her, but as he was doing so another girl fell and dragged the rope with her. Russell adopted a prone position in an attempt to stop the plunge, but all seven climbers on that particular rope disappeared over the bluff. They fell 40 feet before continuing to slide down the Maketawa Valley. Some travelled for nearly 400 yards into the narrow, rock-strewn recess.

In the moments leading up to the plunge, the rasp of Keith Russell's ice axe on the frozen snow was the only sound, as the wind temporarily died. Then Russell's party fell over the bluff and an uncanny silence descended. Quickfall, who had witnessed the accident, made his way as quickly as he could to the Tahurangi Hut and raised the alarm. Back in 1953 communications were basic. Today a rescue helicopter can be summoned in fifteen minutes and climbers in trouble can be plucked off a mountain inside an hour. In the Tahurangi Hut there was just one phone and it wasn't possible to summon everyone in good time to realise an immediate rescue. This was the era when messages were flashed on cinema screens to summon rescuers in the event of mountain dramas.

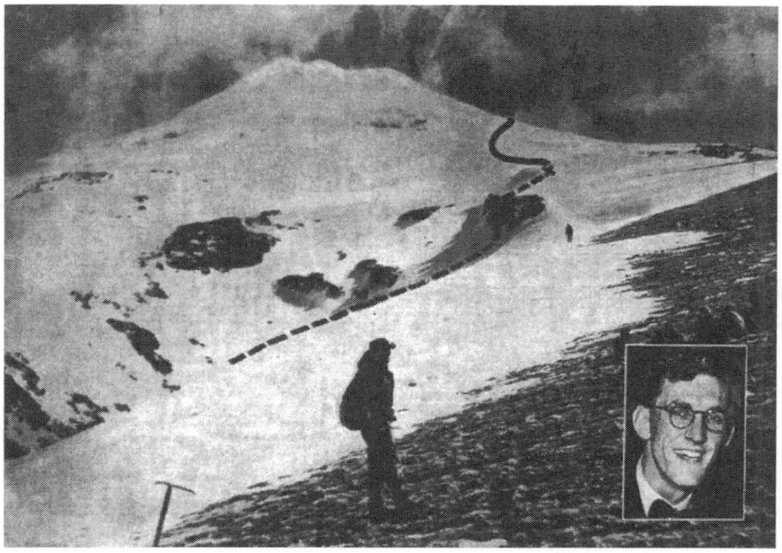

Newspaper coverage of the accident. An X marks the point where the climbers fell, the dotted line the direction of the fall. Keith Russell is shown in the inset photo. (The auckland Star)

Nonetheless, the police were telephoned and the Alpine Club's search and rescue organisation activated. Members of the latter climbed rapidly to the accident site. Four victims were found roped together near the foot of Hongi's Bluff. Two more were located further down the mountain and the seventh several hundred yards from Hongi's Bluff.

The conditions confronting the rescue team were challenging. The weather had deteriorated further and blizzard conditions prevailed. Working in total darkness took a rare degree of bravery. Would it be a case of someone needing to rescue the rescuers? Torches came into their own when the moon disappeared behind the clouds. Even when the moon shone, it cast eerie shadows making rescue attempts more difficult.

Ironically, the blizzard made some things easier for the rescue team, for the freshly deposited soft snow made the icy slopes less dangerous. However, injured victims of the accident suffered terribly, and although four alpine club members tried to keep them warm, there was quite a wait for stretchers to be carried up the mountain.

By now the centre of rescue operations had been transferred to the Nissen Hut. It was decided to move the victims there, as it was only half a mile from the accident site. Accordingly medical supplies and other provisions were moved from the Tahurangi Hut. A fire was lit in the Nissen Hut and beds warmed with heated stones and hot-water bottles.

In all, about 100 people participated in the rescue. Despite such numbers it was still close to midnight before the first stretchers reached Nissen Hut. It must have been an ordeal easing the victims off the mountain in such unforgiving conditions. As the victims arrived at the hut, most were found to have head injuries and broken bones, not to mention a fair degree of exposure.

From the Nissen Hut the victims were moved to North Egmont Hostel. It wasn't until midmorning of the following day that this exercise was completed. It was sobering to the rescuers when they learned that only two casualties made it to the North Egmont Hostel alive. When one of these also died in hospital the next day, the rescuers had to come to terms with the fact that six climbers were dead. The only survivor was a woman who had suffered a broken leg.

Taranaki was shocked by the incident, and New Plymouth in particular, for the four deceased nurses had worked at the local hospital. They were members of the Nurses Tramping Club and it was immediately said that climbing Mt Egmont was not exactly tramping. A strong whiff of irresponsibility emerged early on. It was doubly galling at the time that four of the six victims should be women. This was in the age when the 'girls can do anything' mantra hadn't emerged and males were expected to be protective of women. The first serious accident involving a woman on Mt Egmont had occurred in 1913 when Evelyn Oxenham, aged 22, from Fitzroy, died from exposure. Men were castigated over that death, too.

Some remarked that Egmont was seen as an easy scramble for hundreds in summer, yet often in winter became an icy climb requiring high technical standards. It seemed that only the positive aspects of that sentiment hit home. The dangers of winter climbing were less earnestly expressed. In fact, winter mountain climbing in New Zealand has always been fraught with danger.

Even today, hardly a week passes without the news media advising us of someone losing their life on a mountain. Often such accidents are caused by sudden changes in weather patterns in mountainous environments. The Mt Egmont tragedy featured dramatic weather shifts. What started out as a perfect day, with clear blue skies and a light, cool breeze from the southeast, turned into something decidedly different once the party had reached the summit. Conditions deteriorated dramatically and the south-easterly breeze became a strong wind gusting to forty knots. However, there were other factors unrelated to the weather to consider.

The Mt Egmont tragedy featured dramatic weather shifts.

At the inquest in New Plymouth, the District Coroner was quite categorical about the part played by the Taranaki Alpine Club – or rather the part that wasn't played. Inexperienced climbers had asked the club to help them in their endeavour, to provide guidance in their expedition to get to the top of Egmont and back. Whether a cavalier attitude by the males of the Alpine Club towards the nurses was part of the problem, or whether it was simply a communication breakdown that led to inadequate instruction and slipshod safety advice, it was generally accepted that the accident was the result of non-adherence to the tenets of safe mountain climbing.

Attitudes and poor communication may have been significant factors, but on a more practical level, the equipment provided for the novice climbers probably told a story. Of the larger party that set out on that fateful day only Keith Russell, the experienced climber, and Dick Williams, a comparative novice of the

Taranaki Alpine Club, were wearing crampons. A further 20 climbers had ice axes, but the eleven nurses involved were allocated single ski poles only. A pecking order seemed to be a component of the expedition.

The sad affair became known as the 'nurses' accident'. The *Taranaki Daily News* pointed out that it was New Zealand's worst alpine tragedy. Six climbers on Mt Egmont fell to their deaths in unearthly silence. Keith Russell, Andrew Lornie, Ruth Caldwell, Janet Cameron, Julie Cassells, Ellen McBeth and Ann Tomlinson slipped over the edge of Hongi's Bluff. All but Tomlinson died.

With the benefit of hindsight, perhaps it can be suggested that New Zealanders in the 1950s, moving away from the shadows and strictures of the war years, were inclined to be a little less cautious than they should have been in some of their outdoor activities. They may have been throwing caution to the wind after all the negativity and denial of the period 19391945. Or was it simply a matter of people underestimating Mt Egmont and its potential danger?

How else do you account for a second tragedy on Egmont little more than a week later? Two young men died on the mountain soon after dusk. Mystery surrounded their deaths. Locals began looking sideways at their mountain.

21

THE TRAGEDY OF THE ROYAL MUSTANGS

The crash of two formation fighters 1953

They say the North American P-51 Mustang is quite easy to fly. Talk to flying enthusiasts or private pilots and you will find that to fly one is a common fantasy. Designed, built and flown in 183 days in mid-1940, rakish and good looking, the Mustang had a top speed of .76 Mach, or 76 per cent the speed of sound – equal to the Strikemaster jet manufactured several decades later.

In August 1945, thirty crated Mustangs arrived in New Zealand under the lend-lease arrangement with the US, but with the cessation of hostilities, they were placed in storage near Auckland. In 1952 a decision was made for them to be assembled and supplied to the Territorial Air Force. The Territorial pilots, engaged under the Compulsory Military Training scheme, could be people who normally worked in any civilian occupation. At training camps they would attract envious glares as they taxied about, canopy slid back, arm resting casually on the fuselage as if they were driving a sports car about to pick up girls.

By 1955 many of these aircraft had developed corrosion problems and the decision was made to scrap and dispose of the Mustangs. Wings severed by blowtorch, the dismembered hulks typically attracted a bid of around £70. However, one buyer was able to acquire compatible parts from a paddock near Motueka, where a complete wing and undercarriage assembly had escaped the torch. After several years of rebuilding effort, an airworthy Mustang emerged. Once it had been test flown, the owner nudged the test pilot and asked if he 'could have a go'. Thus Auster pilot became Mustang pilot, flying in and out of a large paddock in Aylesbury without incident. In the 1990s, anyone could pay for a ride in a Wanaka-based Mustang with controls in the back and execute effortless aerobatic rolls from the back seat.

In December 1953, New Zealand became immersed in a royal love affair, when the stunning Princess Elizabeth, who had recently become Queen, made the very first visit by a reigning monarch to New Zealand. She arrived on the Royal Yacht *Gothic* on 23 December 1953. As part of the royal welcome, a formation of RNZAF Mustangs was to fly overhead that morning. On the preceding day, four Mustangs were to be flown from Ohakea to Whenuapai. The leader of the formation was Squadron Leader Maxwell Barrington Stevens, aged 34, and his second-in-command was Flying Officer Richard Maurice

Westrupp, aged 28, both of Wellington. They were regular Air Force pilots, while Flying Officer Lawson in number 3 and Flying Officer Scott in number 4 were Territorial pilots.

On the morning of 22 December the weather was not good, with a stationary front lying across the central North Island. At Ohakea the cloud ceiling was 1000 feet with four to five miles visibility, suitable for departure later in the afternoon provided precautions were taken against deteriorating weather conditions en route. It was decided to follow the coast around Cape Egmont in finger four formation; that is, leader in front, number 2 and number 3 spaced out behind each wingtip, with number 4 behind and to the right or left of number 3 as determined by such things as coastline or terrain. The flight was under Visual Flight Rules (VFR), meaning minimum visibility of three miles, clear of cloud and with ground surface below the aircraft in sight at all times. This would, for example, preclude flight in or above cloud. Experienced VFR pilots tell you that in bad weather the safest place to be is on a coastline following a line of surf. They say the line of surf stands out almost as if illuminated.

The VFR flight plan submitted to Air Traffic Control advised a true airspeed of 280 knots, following the coast. At the briefing the pilots were told to fly a close formation, but if they ran into bad weather they were to fall back into line astern. It was also mentioned that if by chance they had already run into bad weather they would be given instructions over the radio to lower flap and reduce speed. They were briefed that if the weather deteriorated further and it became necessary for the leader to make fairly tight turns in order to keep the coast in view, the formation was to spread out. It was understood that all were to proceed independently if visual contact was lost.

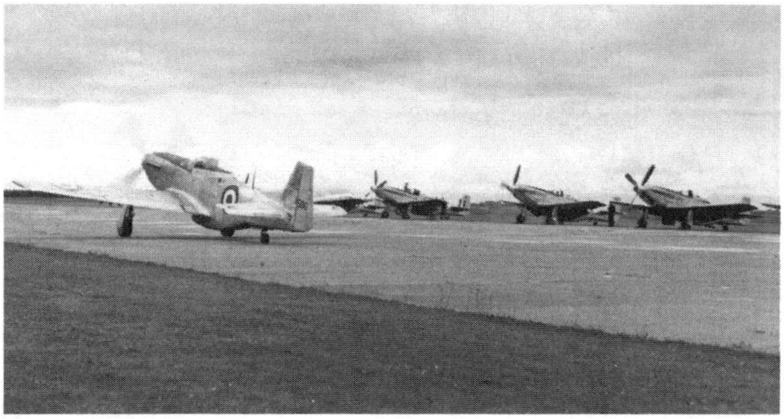

Operational for just three years in the 1950s, the RNZAF Mustang was much loved, but almost half of them were destroyed in accidents. (Alexander Turnbull Library, P51D 63889 1/2)

After the formation took off at 3.11p.m., cloud base and visibility diminished steadily as they proceeded around Cape Egmont, and by the time they reached New Plymouth, where the airport was closed, conditions were below VFR limits. Flying past the airport at 150 feet, the leader did not respond to a call from the control tower asking if they were coming in to land. At this point number 3 was losing sight of number 1 and number 2, who both eventually disappeared behind a bank of coastal fog near Urenui, so to catch up, number 3 boosted his power setting, regaining 210 knots. Number 4 was 200 yards behind and to the left of number 3 when at 3.50p.m. and 20 miles north of New Plymouth, he too lost sight of the aircraft in front of him. Following instructions, he lowered flap, reduced speed to 170 knots and turned slightly out to sea, allowing a widening gap to grow between 3 and 4. He then heard the leader call 'all those still with me please answer in turn.' Expecting number 2 to call first, number 4 did not answer straight away but after a few moments called his leader to say he was proceeding independently, as briefed. There was still no reply from number 2. Number 3 thought the leader had said something about turning and asked for clarification, then replied that he too was breaking formation and, turning slightly to the left, flew on at high speed a few feet above the waves. The leader acknowledged both calls, and his last words were 'it's pretty thick here but we will press on.'

Nobody knows for certain what happened next, but at 4.10p.m. Tongaporutu farmer Walter Burton heard a rapidly intensifying noise and was suddenly confronted by the terrifying spectacle of a Mustang bursting low through the fog at such a speed there must surely be a catastrophic crash. His teenage son Richard was 100 yards away but could not catch sight of the Mustang before fog swallowed it completely. The engine cut, as if the pilot was trying to see the ground beneath, then revved up suddenly. There was a heavy thud, then the unmistakeable sound of exploding high octane gasoline. Following the direction of the noise, Richard Burton ran into the bush and soon spotted the burning wreckage. His father rang New Plymouth control tower to report the crash at 4.37p.m.

On reaching Tirua Point, well to the north, at 4.00p.m., F/O Scott called his leader asking if they should get a weather report from Whenuapai, but the leader did not reply. At one point F/O Lawson recalled that his altimeter was indicating 150 feet and he still could not see the surface of the water, and at another stage he had to turn sharply to avoid striking some cliffs. Shortly after this, weather conditions improved slightly enabling 3 and 4 to climb back up to 1000 feet and continue normally to Whenuapai, where they touched down at 4.33p.m. and 4.45p.m. respectively. Dismounting, Lawson and Scott were presented with the grim news that one of their formation had crashed and another was missing. They retired to the mess where they awaited developments and made debriefing statements.

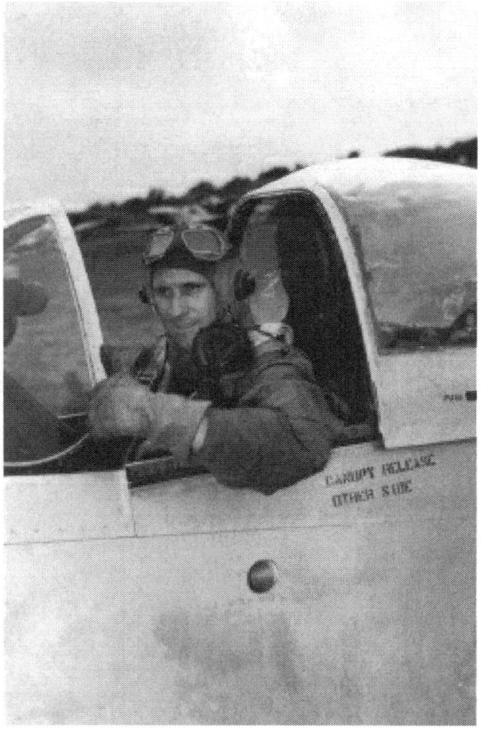

In 1953 most telephone exchanges throughout New Zealand hosted party lines, that is, several subscribers had a shared connection and the system was manually operated. Thus electrifying news was transmitted at human speed. Calls back to a Flight Lieutenant at Ohakea revealed that he was expected home at 6.05. Repeated calls to the officers' mess at Shelly Bay failed to locate an urgently needed chaplain. Numerous calls to the Minister of Defence were not picked up. The wife of the president of the Federation of Mountain Clubs politely told frantic callers that her husband was not in. But by 6.00p.m. the calls were starting to gain traction. News that fuel reserves of the missing Mustang would have run out by 6.10p.m. galvanised sterner effort.

By 6.45p.m. Search and Rescue was swinging into action and shortly thereafter, accompanied by police, they descended on the Burton property. Everyone clung to the hope that the pilots might have baled out. Either or both might be in the sea or wandering dazed and confused on a beach. The wife of one of the pilots enquired whether a launch was being put out. The fate of one Mustang was known, but the second one might have climbed above cloud and come down anywhere at all. Search logistics were mind-boggling. Overnight, the police arranged for a sombre message to be read out repeatedly over 2YA radio: 'Information is sought on the whereabouts of one Mustang of RNZAF missing between Ohakea and Auckland. Was with party of four Mustangs that passed over Waitara at 3.50p.m. today. Any person having any information of this aircraft is required to contact the police immediately.' To cope with responses, all telephone exchanges throughout the country were required to be staffed throughout the night, a considerable undertaking as most normally shut down at midnight.

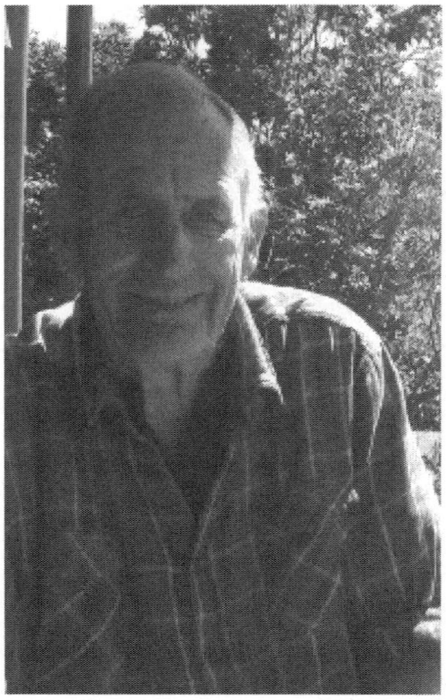

Richard Burton in 2014, the last surviving witness to the Mustang crash of December 1953. (Russell Young)

The next day, as rescuers struggled to excavate the red-hot wreckage, reports of sightings came in. An instructor at Wanganui reported seeing the formation flying at 150 feet towards Patea at 4.00p.m. A farmer at White Cliffs said he saw one travelling north very fast and very low. He said that moments later another came past 'too close' to the cliffs, and he heard the engine noise die suddenly. A workman at Mohokatino had seen two Mustangs heading north just above the sea at 4.50p.m. Walter Burton said he heard another Mustang moments after the crash, apparently flying out to sea, then heading south and then north. A traffic officer at Waitara had seen one coming from an easterly direction, pass low overhead, then turn north tracking up the coast, when the engine noise died suddenly in the distance. He claimed his time of just before 4.00p.m. was 'definite'. Several people north of Mokau reported seeing two Mustangs a few minutes apart flying north very fast, 30 feet above the waves.

At the crash site, rescuers refused to give up hope that the pilot may have baled out. Grim excavation efforts were slowed by the hot metal parts, and nullified by trees and loose soil that kept falling back in. Service personnel were joined by amateur radio operators to pass messages using war-surplus 48 sets and ZC1s, but a squabble broke out between them as the amateurs were still using a superseded phonetic alphabet. Inaccuracies in the new mosaic photographs briefly led searchers to believe that both wrecks had been found, with this misinformation entering and then clogging the entire message system. Having toiled all day, rescuers finally found the remains of the pilot at 5.00p.m. and identified the wreckage as NZ2404, piloted by Squadron Leader M. B. Stevens.

The search for the second Mustang consumed five more days, until a farmer at White Cliffs, acting on a hunch, drove along the beach at low tide and found wreckage in a stream bed. The Mustang had dug a hole 20 feet deep and so sheer that two search parties had traversed within 100 yards without spotting it. The wreckage was still too hot to touch and the body of pilot Richard Westrupp was not recovered until the following day.

The Mustang had dug a hole 20 feet deep

The Court of Enquiry pondered the various reports, but as there had been no witnesses to the second crash, had to conclude that the most likely cause was that the pilot of each aircraft lost control in fog while attempting to avoid collision with terrain. The possibility of a mid-air collision may have been considered but was not stated in the report. Some aspects of the sightings did not seem to reconcile. As both 3 and 4 were well north by 4.00p.m., which Mustang was seen by the Waitara traffic officer? Was this perhaps number 1, worried about number 2, circling back to have a look, then striking peril very close to the spot where number 2 disappeared? How reliable was the time of crash? The Wanganui instructor and the Mohokatino workman both seemed to be one hour out with their times.

Several books state mid-air collision as the cause, despite the findings of the Court of Enquiry. But Tongaporutu locals are sure. They know. It was, after all, their disaster. It is as if they own it, which in a way they do: the two wrecks are still in the ground just eight miles apart, evidence enough, surely, of a mid-air collision. Timing of the various sightings, they say, is too unreliable to conclude otherwise. Richard Burton was still alive in 2014 and could clearly recall what he saw and heard the day of the crash.

Today, when the fog comes down on the Tongaporutu coast, locals still call it 'Mustang weather'.

22

THE WEEPING WATERS

The Tangiwai rail disaster 1953

The year 1953 was a momentous one for New Zealand and its inhabitants. Eight years after the conclusion of the World War Two hostilities, we had learnt to forget the worst aspects of the global conflict. We were basking in the glow of the 'golden weather' years when Kiwis knew their place and social mayhem was a largely unknown concept. You could leave your doors unlocked and not just the back one. Men brought home the bacon. Women cooked it and had babies. Towns and suburbs were glued together by mothers in days when women going out to work were uncommon.

Prosperity was on the rise too, so much so that some single-income families could afford to buy their own car. Not that railways suffered much as a result in the early 1950s. Expresses and limiteds, railcars and mixed trains ran all over the national network. It was the way we travelled, both long distance and locally.

It had been a golden year. An unknown bee-keeper named Edmund Hillary had become the first man to climb Mount Everest, an unheard-of feat. The All Blacks, who had up-ended the British Lions in 1950 and in 1951–52, had played Australia five times and only a single defeat had besmirched their record. The memory of that wretched 1949 season when the All Blacks somehow managed to lose all six tests was well and truly buried. And now the All Blacks were off on their grand tour to Britain and France.

To top it all off, the new young Queen Elizabeth, crowned earlier in 1953, was touring among us with her dashing husband, the Duke of Edinburgh. There were very few anti-royalists to express their opposition. Most New Zealanders were pro-establishment and conservative at heart.

New Zealand Railways were conservative too – and reliable. They may not always get you where you wanted to go on time, but they always came through. They were as solid as the All Blacks. As solid as the pies and rock cakes sold at refreshment rooms up and down the line. Nothing flash, really. You could travel first class or book a sleeper, but most egalitarian Kiwis opted to join the throng in the second-class carriages.

And throngs they were. On one famous night during this era eight expresses, relief expresses, limiteds and relief limiteds left Wellington heading for Auckland. The same number left Auckland in the opposite direction. You couldn't help but feel that half the nation was on the move by rail on that remarkable night.

On Christmas Day 1953, we learned that New Zealand had suffered a very serious train crash. The Wellington to Auckland express had fallen into a flooded river after a bridge collapsed, and many people were dead.

The link between the crater lake on Mount Ruapehu and New Zealand's worst rail disaster was little known to most. Yet the connection was not a revelation to some people. After all, nearly thirty years earlier the sudden erosion of the crater lake had led to the release of vast amounts of water down the nearby Whangaehu River, across the plains, and beneath the rail bridge that had been built to ford the Whangaehu at a tiny locality called Tangiwai.

The wave of 1925 was estimated to be six metres high, virtually the same as the wall of water that struck the rail bridge in 1953, causing sufficient undermining and damage to render the bridge impassable. In 1953 the Wellington to Auckland express – or a significant part of it – plunged into the raging torrent from the crater lake and 151 people lost their lives. It was New Zealand's worst rail disaster.

In 1925 the bridge had suffered damage but it had held together sufficiently to allow the passage of trains, albeit at a slow and cautious pace. Meanwhile, repair gangs reinforced the bridge and for months afterwards trains crawled across it. The damage had obviously been significant.

The link between the lahar – the sudden flash flood of crater-lake water – and the rail bridge had made its presence felt before. Even before there was a railway the phenomenon had been witnessed and recorded. Away back in the mid-nineteenth century, another such flood destroyed the existing road bridge across the Whangaehu. It was described as a wall of milky white water from the lake when the crater had filled and couldn't physically contain the build-up anymore. The collapsing wall carried huge chunks of ice and snow with it in a slurry of diluted sulphuric acid from the volcano. Great boulders and massive tree trunks were swept along by the force of the outpouring.

In less than three hours the freak flood had run its course, out to the Tasman Sea, leaving a trail of boulders, massive ice chunks, tree trunks, bridge timbers and other debris. Everything smelt of sulphur, and even compacted ice and snow were black in colour. On a hot summer's day, the muddy ice strewn across the land melted slowly, sending off an eerie vapour that took on the resemblance of smoke. It must have been a bizarre spectacle.

It can be assumed that the flash flood or lahar that caused so much damage and heartache on Christmas Eve 1953 resembled the midnineteenth century one, although there would have been few people in that sparsely populated part of the North Island who witnessed the surge in 1953. The disaster occurred under cover of darkness. Several witnesses heard the roar of the flood though, but attributed it to other phenomena – natural or otherwise.

A shocking number of New Zealanders were washed away, many forever.

For a nation to have to endure a major disaster at any time is mortifying. For it to occur on Christmas Eve was doubly horrifying. After the announcement a sense of disbelief descended. A shocking number of New Zealanders were washed away, many forever, the victims of a flash flood that came out of a clear blue sky on the day before Christmas. It hadn't even been raining, so how could flooding have occurred? Many Kiwis were mystified.

Over the next few days Kiwis learned as much as they wanted to know about lahars – flash floods of mud and rock – and the link between two national icons, one natural, one manmade: Mount Ruapehu and its crater lake, and the North Island Main Trunk railway line. At 10.21p.m. the Wellington to Auckland express skewed off the weakened bridge. Engine KA 949 and the first five second-class carriages disappeared into the maelstrom. The sixth carriage, the first of the first-class cars, hovered on the rim of the now gaping river bridge before it, too, slipped over the edge.

There were 285 passengers on the train. Eight passengers left the train at Waiouru, the last stop before the disaster site. One passenger climbed on board.

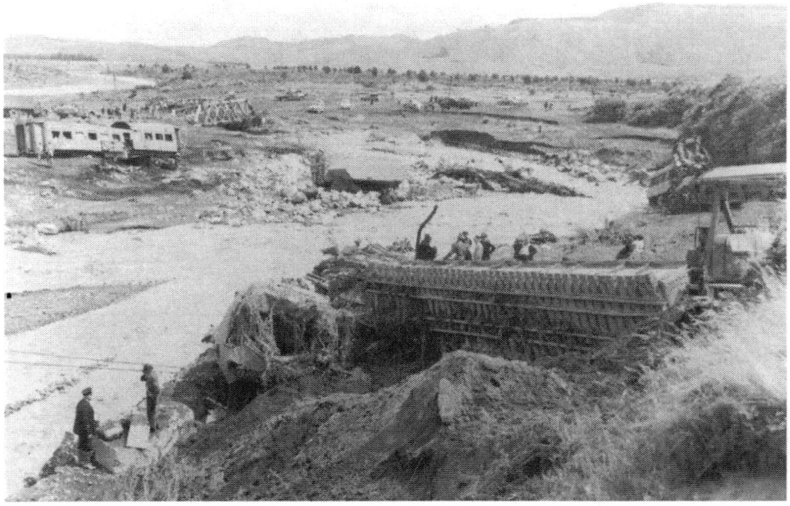

The scene of utter desolation following the lahar at Tangiwai.
(Alexander Turnbull Library, Ref: EP/1953/2617-F)

That evening Cyril Ellis happened to be driving from Taihape across the Tangiwai road bridge and realised the danger to the approaching train. He ran down the railway track towards the train brandishing a torch, in the hope that the driver or fireman would see his light and have time to stop the express. Despite his efforts, the express plunged into the river.

The train was halfway across the bridge when it buckled, and the engine nosedived into the torrent. The first carriage remained connected to the engine, the second broke free and pulled the next three carriages into the flood.

Some of the carriages were badly damaged, others remained remarkably intact and produced many survivors. Two carriages were propelled by the surge across the adjacent main road. One was carried two kilometres downstream. Three carriages were rammed up against the river banks.

Many passengers were trapped in the swirling carriages and drowned. Some of those who were thrown free into the river were able to swim to safety. Others were simply swept to safety. Some were able to smash their way clear of the carriages, only to be taken by the muddy, sulphurous waters, now engorged with oil from the ruptured tanks of the engine. Some died after becoming snarled in gorse bushes downstream, while others were swept away by the angry waters and their bodies were later found many kilometres away. The power of the flood could be attested to by the fact that some bodies were never accounted for and it was likely they had been swept out to sea, 120 kilometres from the Tangiwai bridge site.

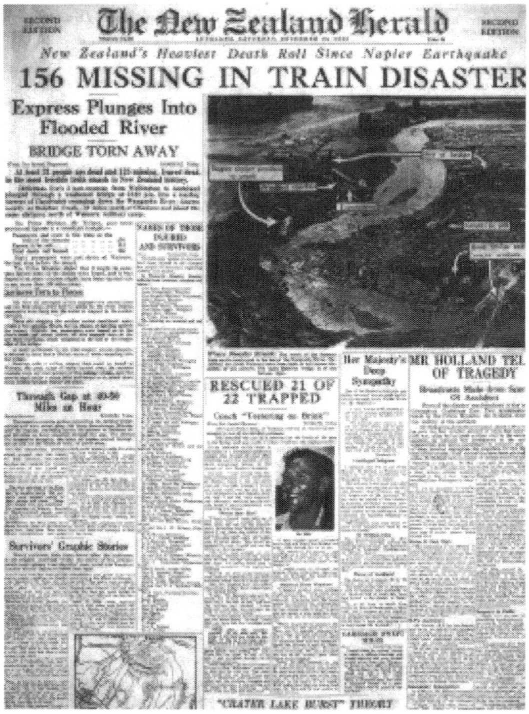

The New Zealand Herald

New Zealand's Heaviest Death Roll Since Napier Earthquake

156 MISSING IN TRAIN DISASTER

Express Plunges Into Flooded River

BRIDGE TORN AWAY

RESCUED 21 OF 22 TRAPPED

Her Majesty's Deep Sympathy

MR HOLLAND TEL OF TRAGEDY

Typical newspaper coverage of the Tangiwai disaster, December 1953. (New Zealand Herald)

There were some remarkable tales of survival. In the carriage directly behind the engine two groups of four survived. A Dunedin family found a broken window in time, through which they all crawled to safety. The other group – four men playing cards – met up, all in one piece, on the river bank. Their recollection of how they got there was less lucid. They found it hard to believe that they'd all survived.

Another carriage landed on its wheels and the windows fell open. While this enabled the putrid water to rush in, it also assisted passengers to get out. Once they'd clambered through the windows, several managed to cling to the roof which was protruding about nine inches above the flood. Eventually they made it to the river bank.

While the disaster raged, staff at the Waiouru Military Hospital were putting up the last of the Christmas decorations and enjoying a festive party when news of the calamity first got through. The dispatches were sobering, and before long rescue teams sped towards Tangiwai. The hospital was made ready to receive the many injured passengers. Significantly there were few injuries to tend. The nature of the disaster meant that those with injuries were at a disadvantage against the surging flood and were invariably swept to their deaths. In the end, 21 received treatment at Waiouru Hospital, 12 at Raetihi Hospital and 12 at the small Forestry Service camp at Karioi.

The heartrending search for victims' bodies continued. Official search parties were complemented by over 100 nearby farmers and townsfolk. As the water receded, bodies were found amongst the willows on the river bank. A considerable distance from the crash site a woman was found buried up to her neck in mud and silt. She was alive and uninjured.

As more and more bodies were found, they were transferred to the Waiouru Army Camp's social hall. Soon the dance floor was covered with coffins and sheeted bodies. Most of the victims were without clothing, a result of the incredible force of the floodwaters. Eventually trains left the area, taking the dead home in wagons marked with large white crosses. Unidentified corpses were carried to Wellington where a special funeral service attended by the Duke of Edinburgh was held.

Soon the dance floor was covered with coffins and sheeted bodies.

It wasn't until the following April that the final official death toll was released. Of the 285 people known to be on the train, 134 were confirmed as being safe. Bodies recovered and identified totalled 123. Bodies recovered but not identified amounted to eight. Twenty people were never accounted for.

Earlier on that fateful Christmas Eve, a bus driver from the town of Bulls was having a few problems with his passenger bus on the run between Bulls and Turangi. When the radiator came to the boil, he clambered down towards the Whangaehu River with a can to get water to ease his radiator's plight. Before he knew it, the Whangaehu was suddenly at his feet rushing past at a rate of knots. Apart from the untoward speed of the flow, the colour and consistency of the water was startling. It was thick, grey and contained black specks and rocks.

Obviously the crater lake lahar was already in motion, and rather than curse the lack of conventional fresh water for his bus radiator, the driver should have sensed danger. Perhaps he didn't know about the destructive force of such a rare event. After all, it wasn't every day that the crater lake burst its confines. But there had been evidence of such flash floods before – sufficient to convince the railways that some warning device or safety programme should have been instigated. It seemed as though the potential danger had been swept under the carpet, and if railway engineers were blasé about the situation, why would a Bulls bus driver worry?

Lewis Vause and Jim Mason were mountaineers and canoeists. They had often climbed Mt Ruapehu, and as canoeists on the crater lake they were alarmed to find that lake levels were rising rapidly. The outcome of such rises had been only too evident over the years. The lake wall would collapse, giving rise to a lahar, which would follow the course of the Whangaehu River to the sea. Vause and Mason warned the authorities in writing of their findings and expressed their concerns in the years leading up to the tragedy. New Zealand Railways and other official bodies did not act on such information.

Fate is by nature capricious. Often we hear of disasters being avoided by human vigilance or freakish natural happenings. At 7.25p.m. on Christmas Eve 1953, a mixed goods train, with its single passenger carriage at the back of a string of goods wagons, roared across the Whangaehu River at Tangiwai. The river was gurgling to the sea in its normal friendly manner. The weather was slightly overcast but there was nothing to suggest that a storm was brewing. Yet two hours later the Whangaehu was host to a fearsome lahar full of mud, boulders and stripped vegetation.

It was extreme bad luck that the Wellington-Auckland Express hit the river bridge when the evil surge was at its highest level. A freakish act of nature had showed its other hand and because of its singular lack of regularity, it caught New Zealand Railways off guard. Lahars were infrequent things pulsing down the Whangaehu. In fact, they were exceedingly rare. The chances of one breaking free from the shackles of the crater lake and timing its run to coincide to maximum ill-effect with the arrival of an express train full of passengers defied belief. Some suspected that if there was a God – and you had to ponder the issue following the unbelievable fury of the lahar and the fact it was also Christmas Eve, the eve of the birth of the Son of God – then that God was not always merciful.

And why New Zealand? This was Godzone, the greatest little country on earth. The place where people felt safe as houses, with doors left unlocked; where most people said 'hello' and many still waved at trains. How many would be waving now?

We'd had rail fatalities before, but no more than you would expect in a rugged, hilly place with significant rainfall. Several of our hitherto worst rail accidents had occurred because of heavy rain and landslides. How many countries in the world could say they lost 151 of their people (at the time Tangiwai was the worst rail disaster in history) in a railway accident brought about by a freakish, random collapse of a crater lake wall and the ugly thrust of a stinking lahar? Such a rail accident had never happened before – anywhere. It wasn't just uncommon, it was unprecedented.

Two hours after the Tangiwai disaster, the level of the Whangaehu had dropped to a mere one metre above normal flow. Such a level wouldn't harm a fly.

The Whangaehu was known locally as 'Sulphur Creek'. The surrounding locality was named Tangiwai. The English translation of Tangiwai is 'weeping waters'.

23

BATTLING THE 'KAIMAI BREEZE'

The Kaimai air accident 1963

Between the end of World War Two and the mid-1960s, disasters involving commercial aircraft in New Zealand occurred with tragic frequency. In October 1948, a National Airways Corporation (NAC) Electra went down on Mount Ruapehu, killing 13. Six months later, in March 1949, a National Airways Corporation Lodestar misjudged its approach to Paraparaumu Airport and the subsequent crash led to 15 fatalities. In November 1961, an Aero Commander went down on Mount Ruapehu, killing six. A Dragonfly aircraft crashed in Fiordland in 1962, leading to another five fatalities.

When early reports came through that a DC3 Skyliner of the NAC fleet was overdue on a flight from Whenuapai to Tauranga on 3 July 1963, few would have been immediately concerned. The DC3 Dakota was one of the most reliable planes flying the commercial routes of New Zealand.

Flight ZK-AYZ flew out of Auckland's Whenuapai Airport 16 minutes behind schedule at 8.21a.m. At 8.35 it reached 5500 feet. All was in order. The pilot, Captain Len Enchmarch, called Tauranga control tower at 9.04 and gave his flight's arrival time as 9.08a.m., requesting permission to drop from 5500 feet to 4100 feet. This was granted by Tauranga control and Captain Enchmarch confirmed the situation: 'Clear to join Tauranga 4100. Vacating 5500.'

All still seemed in order, but after the captain's announcement Tauranga tower lost all contact with the modified DC3 (named Hastings).

While all of these communications had been carried out in the confines of cockpit and control tower, outside a storm was brewing. The dominant feature of the deteriorating weather was a churning wind. It used to be called the 'Kaimai breeze', a more than mild wind that hammers the Kaimai Ranges west of Tauranga several times in winter. It was not to be underestimated and nor was it – by locals.

Farmers with properties on the flanks of the Kaimais were in the habit of securing their cowsheds and barns with wire, and haystacks exposed in the fields were weighted down with lumps of concrete and other heavy items. Meanwhile the DC3 flew onward into the storm, but weather forecasts, as it later proved, had underestimated the strength of the wind. Clouds were hanging low over the range, making visibility a problem and rain was bucketing down. Severe turbulence buffeted the plane.

The plane was flying way too low in the treacherous conditions.

Workers at the Gordon quarry in the lee of the Kaimai Ranges became aware of the noise of aircraft engines. If the plane intended clearing the Kaimais, it might be out of luck. These were the immediate thoughts of quarry workers. The plane was flying way too low in the treacherous conditions. One of the quarry workers took a particular interest in the low-flying plane.

As the seconds passed the engine noises faded, then the quarry worker heard a low 'woofing' sound before the clamour of the wind and rain returned. Several nearby farmers heard the revving sound of aircraft engines and they were all concerned for the fate of the large plane that seemed to be flying too low if it was trying to clear the hills.

The DC3, caught in a sudden down draught, hit a ridge 100 feet from the top of Mount Ngatamahinuera, the highest ridge in the Kaimai Ranges. It hit a rock face while travelling at its normal cruising speed of more than 150 knots. The concerns of the quarry workers and farmers were sufficient to prompt them to set out on foot towards the area where they figured the plane had come down. A horrible sense of inevitability had settled on the group. They were fairly sure that a plane, and a fairly large one, had come to grief. As early as 9.30a.m. a phone call was made to the local police, who confirmed that the Skyliner flight from Auckland, via Tauranga, Gisborne and Napier to Wellington, was missing.

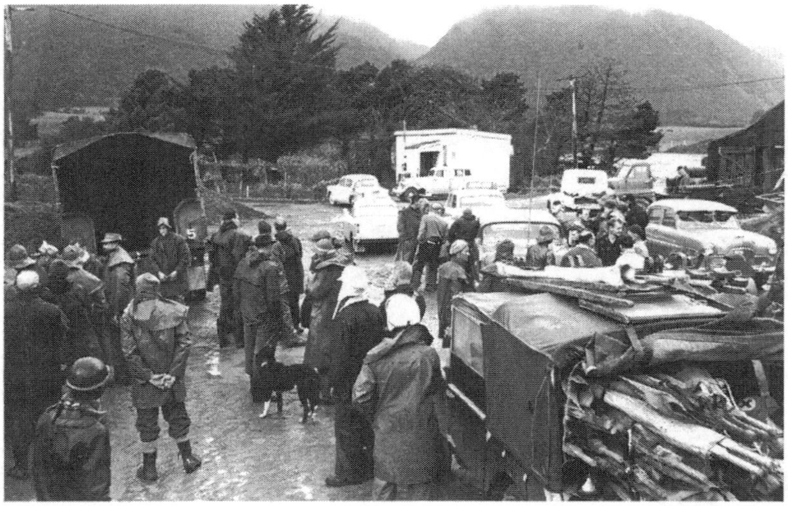

Search parties assemble in the lee of the Kaimai Ranges. (John Charles Collection, Matamata Historical Society)

The search party of locals encountered thick cloud and howling winds as they struggled up the difficult bush- and scrub-clad terrain, and by midafternoon they abandoned the search as the light began to fade. In the end, it took two days to find and reach the crash site, although it wasn't far from the locality of Gordon quarry. By now the army had been called in to supplement the search and rescue effort.

The wreckage was eventually sighted by the pilots of a Bristol Freighter and, based on the information they were able to supply, searchers from a helicopter were lowered to a position below the burnt-out plane. The helicopter pilot had been able to hover fifteen metres above the site, from where he could ascertain that there appeared to be no survivors. The DC3 had hit a rock face, then fallen back into a small pocket of bush below, where it burnt out. All that remained of substance were the tail section and a portion of wing.

The loss of the DC3 Skyliner, and the deaths of all 23 people on board – 20 passengers and three crew – remains the worst air crash to occur in New Zealand. Amazingly, one person survived the immediate crash, only to pass away a few hours later.

As word got around about the disaster, it was often greeted with incredulity. The DC3 was popularly regarded as indestructible. If it had gone down, it would be because of pilot error or extreme weather, certainly not a mechanical malfunction or engine failure. It was unsettling for many to learn that a major air crash had occurred in the Kaimai Ranges. To many Waikato residents, including those living in the lee of the ranges, the Kaimais were the gateway to the golden beaches of Tauranga, Mount Maunganui and further up and down the east coast. Many spent their holidays there in carefree circumstances and it was sobering to consider so much death and destruction occurring little more than a few miles from their summer playground.

The subsequent Court of Enquiry revealed that as well as a severe down draught that made the plane unresponsive, there was also confusion in the minds of the pilots as to where they were located. At one stage the captain announced to the Tauranga tower that he thought he was already east of the Kaimais, when in fact his plane was decidedly to the west. Furthermore, the captain also believed the plane was further along the Kaimais when the crash occurred. The Court of Enquiry found that a significant contributing factor to the crash was the pilot's lack of awareness of his true position, which had instigated an early descent. It was recognised that the pilot only descended to the level officially designated as the minimum safe height.

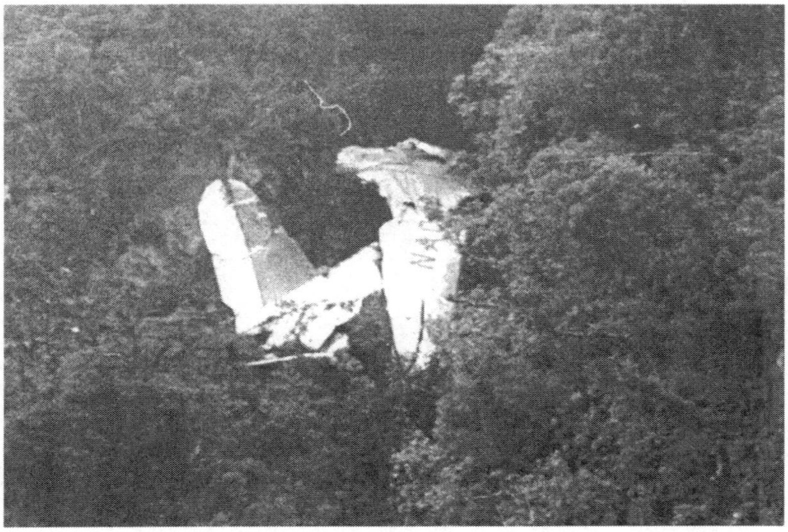

Wreckage of the ill-fated DC3 in the dense Kaimai bush. (John Charles Collection, Matamata Historical Society)

Civil aviation authorities were singled out for classifying the Kaimai Ranges as 'nonmountainous terrain'. Because of this classification, an inappropriate safe altitude for the route was set, and this was identified as another reason for the crash. The classification was later changed.

A lack of technical sophistication at Tauranga Airport was also found to be a factor. The DC3 itself possessed DME (distance-measuring equipment), but this could only be operated if the relevant airport had complementary ground equipment. Tauranga Airport, at the time of the accident, had not been equipped with such equipment. Then it was revealed that the DME equipment on the DC3 was deficient anyway. There had been many pilot reports on the faulty gear.

One of the most telling observations to emerge from the enquiry was the general lack of information about the storm. There was a distinct correlation between stormy weather and troublesome turbulence and down draughts in the region of the Kaimais. During the night of 2 July, the storm had shown its early colours, and power poles were blown over in the Gordon region on the morning of 3 July. Alarm bells should have been rung from that point, yet a revised forecast, taking the storm into account, was not issued until 11.35a.m.

Then there was the misleading forecast of the wind patterns between Whenuapai and Tauranga and the underestimation of the strength of the 'Kaimai breeze'. Perhaps the local rural gift for understatement had caused confusion in the wider world. In truth the 'Kaimai breeze' was nothing less than a howling gale. A large, solidly built community hall at Waiorongomai, an old gold-mining settlement, was bowled over by the 'breeze'. That was near Te Aroha, in the lee of the Kaimais. There should have been a greater urgency relating to the DC3's plight and the danger posed by the wind.

In truth the 'Kaimai breeze' was nothing less than a howling gale.

There was reason to believe that the pilot, through a rare break in the clouds, had seen a township which he took to be Waihi. It was actually Paeroa to the west of the Kaimais. So even at this stage in the fateful flight, the extreme weather conditions had created confusion in the mind of the pilot.

Probably because the Kaimai crash was so serious and so newsworthy, it attracted a certain macabre fascination for rubberneckers, despite the precarious access route to the crash site. Amateur climbers put their own safety at risk as they sought to find the wreckage. As a result, the army was summoned in April of the following year and soldiers blasted away the cliff face in order to bury the remains of the DC3.

It was one thing to literally cover up the physical evidence, but significant litigation went on for several years as the families of the victims sought compensation. For the next of kin, there was no hiding the horror and unexpectedness of the crash.

24

ANY PORT IN A STORM

The sinking of the *Wahine* 1968

Even today, newer generations of New Zealanders find it hard to accept that a vessel as large and seaworthy as the *Wahine* could be thrown around like a child's toy in a bathtub, before sinking with the loss of 51 lives. And if the storm was that bad, how could the authorities have allowed the *Wahine* out on the high seas in the first place?

But no one could have predicted the savagery of the storm that descended on 10 April 1968. What started out as a shallow depression in the Solomon Islands grew very rapidly into a raging hurricane. To compound matters, a cold front approached New Zealand from the south and also developed into a serious storm. The two weather systems met up with each other at Wellington.

On Hawkins Hill near Wellington, winds of 235 kph were recorded. Near Oteranga Bay the winds hit 267 kph. Out at sea, the inter-island ferry *Wahine* was making its way across Cook Strait. Storm warnings had been issued, but Captain Hector Robertson was not unduly concerned. He had helmed the *Wahine* many times between Christchurch and Wellington and the oceans were often as rough as it was in the early hours of 10 April.

As the *Wahine* approached Wellington Harbour the storm intensified. Huge swells and roaring winds made passage more difficult by the minute. Captain Robertson began to feel uneasy. He had never encountered conditions such as this before. The two storm systems had met and all hell was breaking loose. But Captain Robertson trusted his ship to reach the apparent sanctuary of Wellington Harbour.

Just past Pencarrow Heads, the *Wahine* appeared to be on course into the harbour, but then a huge swell twisted her to port by more than 20 degrees. She was now headed for the treacherous rocks of Barrett's Reef. The *Wahine* no longer responded to the helmsman's attempts to get her back on course. She continued to head for Barrett's Reef. A massive wave knocked Captain Robertson off his feet, convincing him that his ship was at the mercy of the rough seas. He made the decision to try and guide the *Wahine* back out of the harbour into Cook Strait.

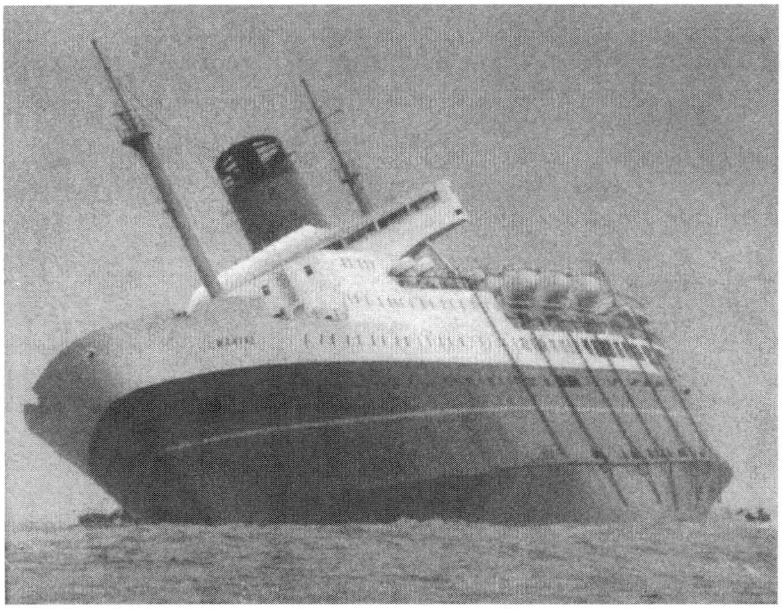

Fatally gashed on Barrett's Reef, the Wahine lists prior to sinking. (Alexander Turnbull Library, Ref: EP/1968/1647/14-F)

The task was made untenable. The radar system was malfunctioning and visibility was virtually nil. Despite Captain Robertson's best efforts, the *Wahine,* with a horrible inevitability, was buffeted on to Barrett's Reef. From that point onwards it became a matter of dealing with the fact that the *Wahine* would, in all probability, sink. It was just a matter of where and when.

Things got worse. Captain Robertson ordered the closing of all watertight doors to reduce the amount of sea water spreading. At this point he heard that the starboard engine was no longer functioning. Very soon the port engine failed too, so both anchors were dropped. The *Wahine* was dragged clear of Barrett's Reef and drifted until the anchors' impact slowed the ship.

There was some encouraging news at this stage. The damage was reported to be serious but not unmanageable. Flooding was found in four compartments. Nonetheless, the order went out to the crew that all lifesaving equipment should be prepared in the event of the situation becoming serious. The *Wahine,* despite losing the battle with Barrett's Reef, was still responding.

But the storm was intensifying. The huge swell increased and now the *Wahine* was dragging its anchors. During this time the passengers had little knowledge of the ship's condition. Most of them were too seasick to truly comprehend the announcement that informed them the vessel was aground on Barrett's Reef. Many had felt the impact as the reef was struck but it had seemed almost inconsequential in the midst of all the noise and pitching and rolling created by the storm. At 8.45a.m. the passengers, now wearing life jackets, were directed to move to B deck.

There were 610 passengers, most of whom were able to assemble in the aft smoke room and the corridors surrounding that section of B deck. The predominant mood was not panic, but boredom. Because the ship was in the confines of the harbour, most considered that the storm would ease, the engines would be powered up and soon they would be berthing. Announcements over the PA system convinced most that they were 'quite safe' and by noon many had taken their life jackets off to use as cushions.

The predominant mood was not panic, but boredom.

The storm continued to rage and visibility was still poor. Attempts were made to attach a line from the tugboat *Tapuhi* to the stern of the *Wahine,* with the intention of pulling the stricken ship towards its destination. However, the line was no match for the power of the storm and the mountainous waves. The line failed.

The *Wahine* was listing badly to starboard now. The outgoing tide was affecting the ship and when she swung around, creating a relatively sheltered environment on the starboard side, Captain Robertson made a fateful call. The bells sounded for 'abandon ship'.

Most passengers were caught off guard. All morning the crew and staff had been reassuring everyone that there was no danger. It later transpired that the reality of the *Wahine*'s plight was kept under wraps in an attempt to prevent panic among the passengers. For more than six hours the passengers had been playing a waiting game, relaxed enough in the knowledge that their life jackets were strictly precautionary.

At the sound of 'abandon ship', many headed for the high port side but there was no chance of using the lifeboats on that side of the ship. Many passengers were disoriented. For nearly seven hours they had been without food. Even if food had been available, the severe seasickness they had been experiencing would have made it unpalatable. And of course they were soon numbed by the stormy conditions. It was little wonder they were unable to carry out basic instructions. Many panicked and found themselves on the raised port side, from where they lost their footing and slid down the deck before crashing into solid objects. Many suffered broken limbs in this manner.

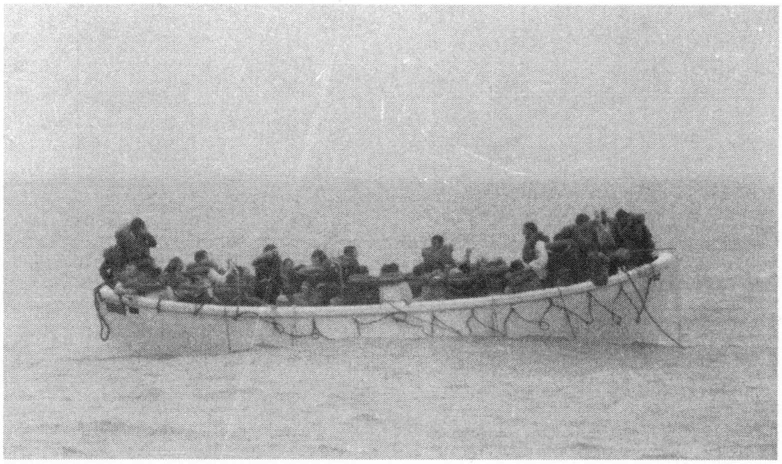

Sodden survivors in a Wahine lifeboat – but they were more fortunate than those left in the water. (Alexander Turnbull Library, Ref: 35mm-01152-29-F)

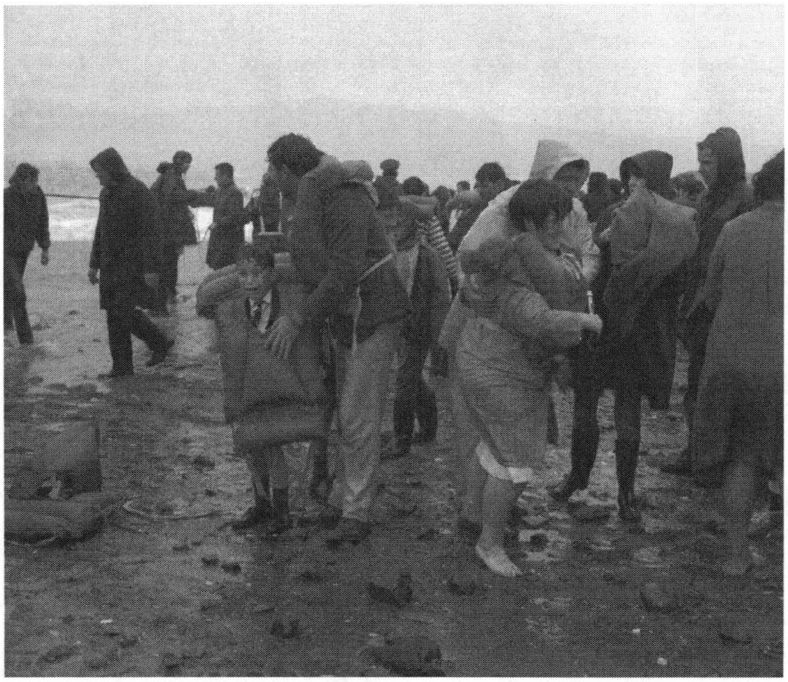

Distraught survivors huddle for warmth following their rescue.
(Alexander Turnbull Library, Ref: EP/1968/1570-F)

Because of the list to starboard, there were only four lifeboats available to take passengers. Seamen attempted to cram as many women and children in them as possible. Most of the lifeboats were swamped by the high seas.

Many people were attempting to move about the boat, but the list and the driving rain made such movements hazardous. Many suffered injuries that were exacerbated by fellow passengers sliding into one another. Older passengers were particularly susceptible, but young children and babies were often separated from their parents as everyone tried to grasp something that wasn't moving.

Panic and fear, held at bay for so many hours, now predominated. Earlier, as long as the *Wahine* was in the confines of Wellington Harbour, most people thought everything was under control, despite the storm. If the boat had drifted out into the wilds of Cook Strait, the passengers may have lost their nerve much earlier.

By now a flotilla of boats and tugboats had been able to put to sea and place themselves where they would be able to pick up passengers who had either jumped directly into the sea or who had been thrown out of life-rafts.

Some passengers, rather than try to find sanctuary in a lifeboat, raft or other craft, took the option of drifting with the mountainous seas towards the Seatoun shore. Some made it. At least they were away from the hulking spectre of the ever-listing ship, threatening at any moment to collapse completely on the starboard side and take out those passengers who had not made it far enough beyond its huge bulk. Some alert passengers, still in the shadow of the listing ship, got hold of wooden planks and were able to use these as paddles to ease life-rafts out beyond the stern of the *Wahine.*

The power of the sea and the perishing cold accounted for many. One lifeboat overturned. Those clinging to the upturned boat steadily became victims of the freezing conditions and fatigue. One by one they lost their grip. Close to 20 were swept away.

Several survivors can remember battling the high seas and cold and losing consciousness somewhere along the line. Their next memory is of waking up on a deserted beach or in the bottom of a rescue vessel. They were the lucky ones. Many of the victims just lost consciousness.

After making a brief search of the decks and lounges to ascertain that there was no one left on board, Captain Robertson and Captain Galloway, the deputy harbourmaster who had earlier joined the crippled ship from the tug *Tapuhi,* dived into the harbour. They were in the water for more than an hour before a launch carried them to safety.

Just before 2.30p.m. two deeply symbolic events occurred at virtually the same time. The *Wahine* slumped to starboard for the last time before coming to rest on the harbour floor. Meanwhile the first of the survivors reached Seatoun. The *Wahine* lay on its side only 400 metres away from the rescuers on Seatoun Beach, and as most of the passengers who came ashore on the Wellington side of the harbour were alive, the enormity of the disaster was still not appreciated.

The* Wahine *lay on its side only 400 metres away from the rescuers on Seatoun Beach.

It was a different matter at Eastbourne on the other side of the harbour. Many bodies were washed up on the rocks and beaches. By the end of the day the number reached 47. Miraculously, 223 survivors had landed on the stretch of coast between Burdon's Gate and Hinds Point on the eastern coast. On the Eastbourne side there was a further impediment to rescue attempts caused by the storm. Several roads were impassable because of slips, and initially only eight policemen were able to reach Eastbourne to assist survivors. Medical teams and rescuers were similarly hampered.

Eventually more than 100 policemen and even more civilian volunteers were able to help the large numbers who came ashore on the eastern side of the harbour. Conditions here revealed the true severity of the disaster. Fifty-one died on 10 April 1968, the day the *Wahine* went down, another died several weeks later and in 1990 a 53rd victim died from injuries sustained in the disaster. All but 12 victims were middle-aged or elderly.

It was New Zealand's worst modern maritime disaster. That it could play out its dramatic hand within the harbour and so close to shore was astounding to many. But then the severity of the storm was such that ordinary practices and perceptions counted for little. The day the *Wahine* foundered has been described as the day New Zealand television came of age. Most of the drama was captured by the cameras and thousands of New Zealanders could see developments from the comfort of their living rooms. Images of the disaster were relayed around the world.

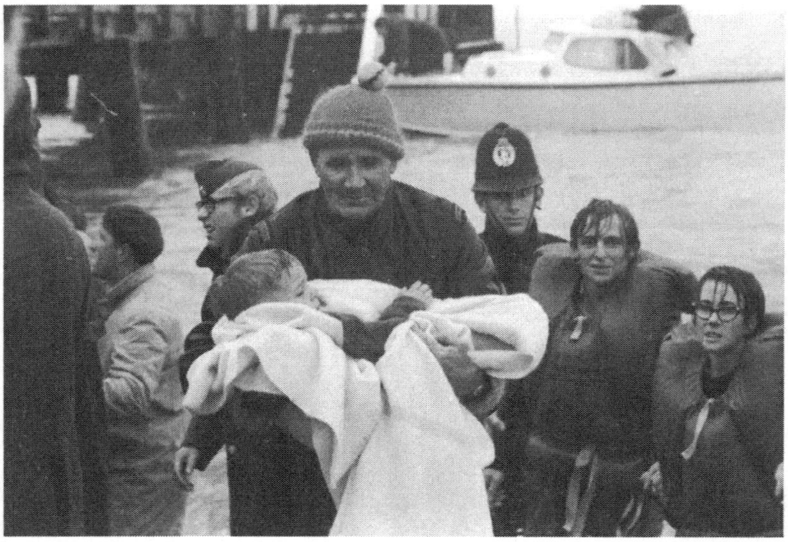

A policeman holds a young survivor of the shipwreck. (Alexander Turnbull Library, Ref: EP/1968/1574/26a-F)

A subsequent Court of Enquiry found faults and omissions in the way the disaster was handled, but did not pinpoint wrongful acts. The extreme weather was the exonerating factor in most situations. Yet the feeling remains that it seemed unnecessary for so many to lose their lives so close to shore.

Watching the *Wahine* list to starboard in Wellington Harbour was surreal. When it capsized the nation gasped. The terrible denouement of the *Wahine's* demise happened under the eyes of the media and thousands of Wellingtonians.

Then the flotilla set out. Too early, some said. Too late, others trumpeted. Owners of launches, fishing boats and other small craft put to sea in an attempt to pick up survivors. Fifty-one people may have died, but it could have been many times worse had the

Wahine succumbed to the lashings of Mother Nature on some lonely coastline miles away from fellow humans with small boats.

New Zealand had known some appalling shipwrecks and foundering in the nineteenth century. The wreck of the *Orpheus* in 1863 produced 189 dead. The *Tararua* disaster of 1881 accounted for 131 fatalities. The *Wairarapa* in 1894 was scarcely less tragic with 121 dead. Those were the serious ones, with the highest mortality totals. There were also hundreds of casualties from lesser shipwrecks.

But that was in the days when most ships were puny wooden structures, set against pulverising seas. What presented itself on 10 April 1968, for much of the world to see, was the demise of a large, modern, ocean-going ferry inside the apparent refuge of one of New Zealand's most significant harbours.

For that reason it was an unusual tragedy, and revealed that the cruel sea, whipped up by the unlikely, hellish confluence of two storm systems, could still play a wicked hand. It was said at the time that if the *Wahine* had not fought the storm, the likes of which New Zealand had never encountered before, for as long as it did, the final death toll would have been markedly different. There may have been only 51 survivors among the 734 souls on board.

25

BLIND FAITH

The Erebus air accident 1979

Drop the word 'Erebus' into any conversation today and within minutes a disagreement may break out. Some will be adamant that the pilots were to blame. Others will be equally vocal in their condemnation of the airline. What they will be discussing is the 1979 air disaster, at that time the fourth largest in aviation history, when 257 people were killed on a sightseeing flight to Antarctica in an Air New Zealand DC10. Some will be supportive of the now famous expression used by the Royal Commissioner appointed to report on the affair, that the airline engaged in an 'orchestrated litany of lies', while others will say the commissioner was incompetent and that this was later proved in a Court of Appeal decision, affirmed by the Privy Council.

The disaster sparked a series of books, all intended to be final and definitive, usually leaning towards one side or the other as to who should bear the blame for the tragedy. Some people will read only those books that support their view, and will stoically refuse to pick up a book that presents an opposite view. The most recent book, stridently in favour of the pilots, was in 2010 by the late Paul Holmes, well known as a journalist and television presenter. His call for a final and formal move by Parliament to exonerate the pilots was quietly declined, on the same grounds adopted by the pilot-error school of thought: the pilots were flying the plane, the plane crashed, end of argument.

Air New Zealand had initiated flights over Antarctica in February 1977 and run them during the summer months. Weekly flights had been taking place in the weeks leading up to the crash. There had been a nationwide publicity campaign with newspaper and television advertisements and publicity brochures delivered to every household. A growing number of passengers had reported by word of mouth the magnificent sights they had seen and exhorted their friends to go. A few weeks before the disaster, there was a news item showing a DC10 cruising at low altitude over the ice. National Film Unit publicity footage taken one week before the crash showed a DC10 disappearing then reappearing behind a low ridge.

Those involved in the disaster bear names that are now well etched into the minds of many: the flight crew, captains Jim Collins and Greg Cassin, flight engineers Gordon Brooks and Nick Moloney, Antarctic commentator Peter Mulgrew, the CEO of Air New Zealand Morrie Davis, chief pilot of the airline Ian Gemmell, chief inspector of air accidents Ron

Chippindale, and the commissioner who headed the enquiry, Justice Peter Mahon. Any mention of these names, even today, may engender feelings of hostility or sympathy and invoke such responses as 'he should have done this', 'he shouldn't have done that', 'he was lying', 'he was incorrect' or 'he was incompetent'.

Inexplicably, in clear air at 1500 feet, it flew straight into the slopes of Mt Erebus.

The aircraft took off from Auckland at 8.20a.m. on 28 November 1979, and by 12.30p.m. was on the threshold of the Antarctic continent with the aim of overflying the spectacular terrain. After descending in two wide orbits to get low enough for sightseeing purposes, the airliner was to proceed down the flat expanse of McMurdo Sound, but instead, inexplicably, in clear air at 1500 feet, it flew straight into the slopes of Mt Erebus, killing all on board. The New Zealand Inspector of Air Accidents was quickly on the case and in due course stated that the probable cause of the accident was the decision of the pilots, who descended below a designated minimum safe altitude and, unsure of their position, continued to fly into an area of reduced visibility and poor horizon definition. While this may well have been factually correct, it raised many more questions than it sought to answer.

At funeral services held up and down the country, some priests implored the mourners to let the matter pass and not engage in a war of blame. The priests pointed out that ultimately everyone could see that the whole concept was dangerous and when people lined up to purchase tickets they knew there could be a risk. A few days after the tragedy, a Sunday newspaper carried a statement from a retired Canadian Air Force pilot with many hours of polar flying experience. He had looked at the maps and could immediately see the ease with which visual landmarks along the intended flightpath could be mistaken in polar conditions. But the official accident report released in March 1980 blamed the pilots completely.

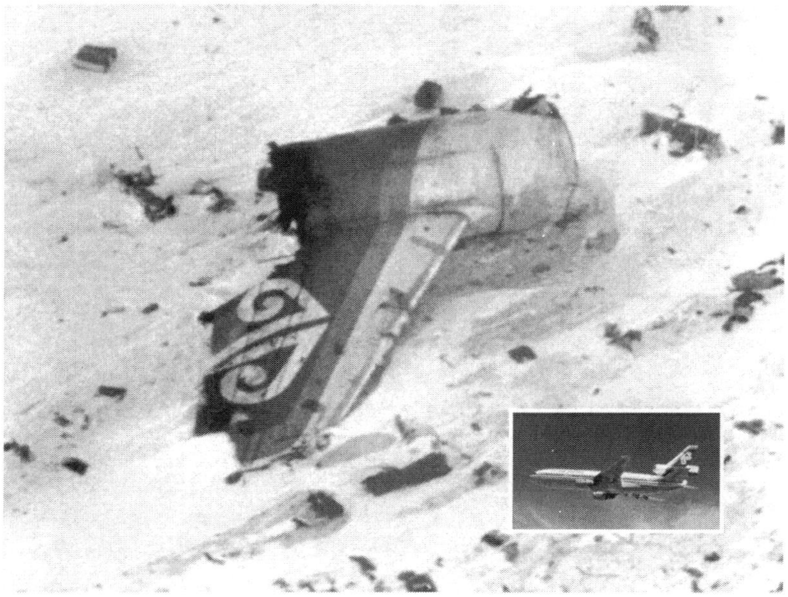

The tail of the DC10 lies in the Antarctic snow. (New Zealand Herald) Inset: A DC10 of similar vintage to the lost plane. (Alexander Turnbull Library, Ref: 1/2-240407-F)

The size of the disaster of course warranted a Commission of Enquiry and a high court judge was appointed as the sole commissioner. The outcome of this led to several years of litigation, followed by decades of controversy. Embittered argument broke out between the Airline Pilots

Flights had indeed been taking place as low as 1500 feet above sea level.

The US base at McMurdo had previously written to the airline outlining the limitations on communication and navigation aids, rescue and emergency facilities, should they ever be needed. It was found that flights had indeed been taking place as low as 1500 feet above sea level, meaning the height over the actual surface could in fact have been much lower. It was found that originally the first few flights had been commenced at 16,000 feet and passed close to the summit of Mt Erebus, which is 11,416 feet high. Another finding was that later flights by the airline had been descending below 16,000 feet, and then below 6,000 feet with assistance from US-manned air traffic control at McMurdo, and had been flying down the flat expanse of McMurdo Sound, sometimes as low as 1500 feet.

It was found that there had been some confusion over the exact coordinates of the waypoint at McMurdo, and that a navigation beacon in McMurdo Sound had recently become unserviceable. Furthermore, a few hours before take-off, essential co-ordinates on the aircraft's onboard computer had not only been changed but in fact contained errors. Where some earlier air crews, and apparently all military air crews, had made it a standard procedure to download and review the co-ordinates loaded into the onboard computer before arrival, such action, if it was carried out in this case, failed to alert the air crew to their ill-fated course.

The Commission of Enquiry was told that, despite a series of recent disastrous technical faults involving DC10s, the DC10 was in fact very safe. It could fly to any point on the globe with stunning accuracy by means of a computerised navigation system. The system was so accurate it almost seemed that the pilots could have stayed in the Koru Lounge and the DC10 could have flown itself to its destination. Ironically, if it had done so it still would have crashed. The pilots could handle polar conditions with ease, using the on-board flight computer to fly accurately between nominated waypoints: recent flights proved this.

Grounds for controversy grew alarmingly when the commissioner sought to find credible answers from the airline or from the government accident investigator about the flight computer. The accident investigator told the commissioner he considered the change in computer coordinates had nothing to do with the crash. An airline executive who had retrieved the captain's flight bag initially swore he had not seen it, then later admitted that he had seen it but that it was empty.

The airline told the commissioner their procedures precluded any flight below 16,000 feet, but tens of thousands of New Zealand homes already held a brochure delivered to their letterbox indicating otherwise, and numerous magazine articles certainly disproved this. A lever arch binder containing the pilot's navigation notes and co-ordinates had been retrieved from the crash site, but when it was presented to the commissioner the pages were missing. The commissioner was told the pages must have been destroyed by fire, blown away in the polar wind, or fallen down a crevasse. An airline official later admitted having destroyed the pages as they were soiled with kerosene, an explanation backed up by his wife.

At one point a Civil Aviation official proposed a scenario which, to be true, would have meant that the pilots, together with the flight engineer, had all suddenly and simultaneously become insane moments before the crash. Vast archives of documents in the airline head office were put through a shredder hours after the crash. Other strange events occurred. The homes of both pilots were entered at times unknown by persons unknown and vital flight documents were removed. The contents of the captain's flight bag were never found.

Eighteen months after the disaster, the commissioner delivered his report containing the now famous phrase that he had been forced to listen to 'an orchestrated litany of lies'. Going beyond his brief, he endeavoured to fine the airline. The commissioner's findings were challenged through the court system, resulting in two Court of Appeal decisions, cancelling the fine and confirming that the commissioner had exceeded his brief and infringed natural justice by failing to allow the airline to respond to the allegations. The end of this process was a 1983 decision of the Privy Council confirming the Court of Appeal decisions.

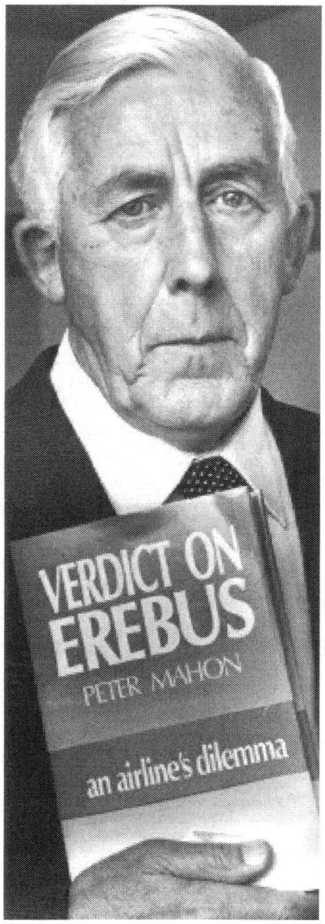

Whatever his findings, Justice Peter Mahon was bound to be criticised. (Alexander Turnbull Library, Ref: EP-NZ Obits-Ma-02)

Further litigation brought by the families of the air crew in 1987 against the US Navy alleging negligence for failure to warn the crew of their dangerous position also failed. While this was the end of litigation, everyone from the Prime Minister down took turns to insult the commissioner. The families of both the airline management and the pilots continued to receive intimidating telephone calls for several years afterwards. Every few months another book would be released on the subject, hoping to settle the matter once and for all.

While the captain on the fatal flight may not have previously flown to the ice, there was always a commentator on the flight deck with knowledge of the area. A number of flights up until 21 November 1979 had been accompanied by a commentator with experience of 57 flights to Antarctica as an observer. He always recommended to the captain of the flight that they circle Mt Erebus before descending. The following week his position was taken by a mountaineer who had considerable experience exploring Antarctica, not by airliner, but on the ground.

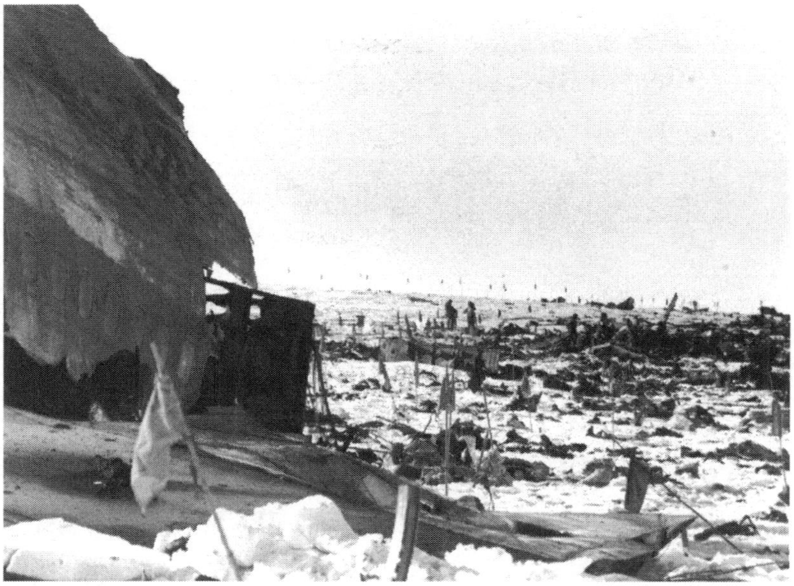

Instant death at the end of the world. It was a tragedy for all New Zealanders. (Colin Monteath, New Zealand Archives, R19892970)

Questions still remained unanswered. Was the airline to blame for allowing inadequately experienced pilots to take passengers to a polar region at low level? Were the computer programmers to blame for having meddled with the flight computer without the flight crew's knowledge? Adjustments had apparently been made to correct reported errors in waypoint coordinates, but the adjustments themselves contained errors. What was the reason for the wholesale destruction of documents by the airline? Were the flight crew to blame for failing to interrogate the onboard computer to ascertain the integrity of the co-ordinates before allowing the computer to take them anywhere? Were the flight crew to blame for declining radar assistance and proceeding at low level into a polar region where the reported conditions would almost certainly result in whiteout and ocular deception, and where the computer was taking the aircraft steadily off track? Thirty years after the disaster, there is still disagreement on many of these issues.

The fact remains that 257 people lost their lives that November day. It was a tragedy that sparked unprecedented national mourning and unparalleled controversy. Maybe the priests at the funeral services for the victims of the disaster were the only ones who were right.

26

A TRIO OF TRAGEDIES

The Marlborough air accidents 1985, 1986, 1996

Between October 1985 and January 1996 three separate air accidents in the Marlborough Sounds claimed a total of 15 lives. All three accidents involved a small aircraft normally engaged in the carriage of passengers across Cook Strait. In two cases there was a lapse of airmanship on the part of the flight crew, and in another a routine maintenance omission led to catastrophic engine failure. Maybe it was these occurrences that gave rise to jokes about flying by 'white-knuckle airlines'. In one case the accident led to the collapse of the airline concerned. As a result of these tragedies, numerous safety procedures were considerably tightened up.

A law change in 1980 permitting competition with established air routes used by Air New Zealand saw the emergence of a number of third-tier airlines, several of which operated in the Cook Strait area. Some, but not all, survived beyond their initial years of operation. Air Albatross initially provided a return service from Nelson to Christchurch and shortly thereafter began a similar service to Wellington comprising several flights a day. On 4 October 1985, commercial pilot Roger Phipps was detailed to fly five flights, beginning at Nelson at 10.30a.m. The first was a ferry flight in a twin-engine Cessna 402 without passengers to Wellington. Rather than climbing to the usual altitude for instrument flight to Wellington, Phipps advised he was descending and would transit by Visual Flight Rules (VFR) through the Marlborough Sounds at low level. He crossed the 2450-ft Maitai Saddle nine miles north-east of Nelson, then followed the Pelorus River to Linkwater, crossing a low saddle into Queen Charlotte Sound near Picton and exiting into Cook Strait through the Tory Channel. This was a 'bad-weather route', well known and used by private and commercial pilots for many years.

In April 1982 the Marlborough Electric Power Board had installed a two-kilometre stretch of three parallel 11,000 volt lines across Tory Channel at Arrowsmith Point, in order to service 30 consumers on Arapawa Island. The maximum height at one pole was 950 feet, extending down to 316 feet in the middle of the span. This aroused considerable opposition in aviation circles, due to the obvious danger presented to aircraft using the bad-weather route.

Safety officials within Civil Aviation agitated in vain against the installation and could possibly have prevented it altogether if they had pointed out that Tory Channel was itself a licensed water aerodrome and no obstruction, such as these cables, could be installed without express approval from the Minister of Transport. But the minister's view was expressed in a letter to one correspondent: 'As Minister, I do not have the power to prevent power lines being erected but may require the owner or person in charge of the project to mark the installations if they are considered to be a hazard to air navigation.'

In response, five orange and white markers were affixed to the wires, a Notice to Airmen (NOTAM) issued, and the location of the span marked on aviation maps with a warning in bold red lettering. But due to an administrative error, the first issue of these maps actually showed the wires in the wrong position. The orange markers were later deemed ineffective and were removed. Aviators were quick to point out that neither the wire nor the spherical markers were visible to a pilot anyway, due to focusing mechanisms in the human eye of a pilot approaching at speed at the same height as the wires. The best option, they said, was not to have the wires there at all.

At midday on the day of the accident the pilot, having recently traversed through the low-level route, asked his passengers if they would prefer to have a flight through the Sounds rather than directly to Wellington over the top of clouds. The passengers included Cindy Mosey, aged 11, her parents Paul and Julie and sisters Karla (13) and Aleisha (7), and another couple, Richard and Dianne Grayson with their 11-year-old daughter Kirsty, all travelling to Wellington for a gymnastics event. The low-level suggestion was enthusiastically taken up by all those on board.

The last radio call from the aircraft was to Wellington Information at 12.09p.m., advising that the flight would be VFR and saying 'actually ... we won't be above 1000 feet.' Several people saw the twin-engine Cessna pass through the Sounds, and at Havelock one witness estimated the height to be between 400 and 500 feet. Nearing Tory Channel, the aircraft banked around, dropping low as it passed over the inter-island ferry *Arahanga* heading to Wellington through Tory Channel. At this point the pilot was turning around talking to his passengers, and crew on the *Arahanga* later testified that the aircraft was low enough for them to see clearly through the windows into the passenger compartment.

At 12.23p.m. the ferry *Aratika* was heading in the opposite direction towards Picton when the crew on the bridge saw the Cessna some distance away flying towards them. The Second Officer was following it through his binoculars saying, 'Gosh, I wonder if she's going under or over the wires' when, with a shower of sparks, the Cessna collided with the cables, broke into several pieces and fell into the sea. The *Aratika* immediately stopped and launched two lifeboats to look for survivors. They were joined by two other vessels nearby. Of the nine occupants, only Cindy Mosey, who had been sitting in the rear of the cabin and had released her seatbelt before final impact, survived, remaining afloat unaided until rescue arrived.

Despite having lost her entire family, Cindy in later life became a sports champion, holding the world title in kite-surfing for three successive years from 2006 to 2008.

The accident investigation found that while the pilot may have been entitled to fly VFR as low as 500 feet in bad weather, he had no need to descend as low as the level of the wires. It criticised airline management for failing to ensure their crews took appropriate steps to remain well clear. Witnesses had observed the aircraft climbing back up as it struck the wires 340 feet above the water.

On the morning of 2 January 1986, a Cessna 207 operated under lease by Skyferry had conducted a flight from Koromiko to the airstrip at Nopera in the Marlborough Sounds without incident. After the engine oil was topped up, the owner himself then resumed control and flew the aircraft back to Koromiko to uplift six passengers for a charter flight to Wellington. With a full load of seven persons, luggage and fuel, the aircraft took off from Koromiko at about 12.40p.m. on runway 36; that is, directly to the north towards the township of Picton. About 90 seconds later several witnesses heard the engine start to run rough and obviously lose power. The pilot had sufficient height to turn around and head back towards the airstrip directly behind him, but when it became apparent they would not make the airstrip, and confronted with a row of power lines along Lindens Road, the pilot attempted another 180-degree turn on to a flat area to his right. The aircraft stalled in the turn and crashed with the loss of all on board.

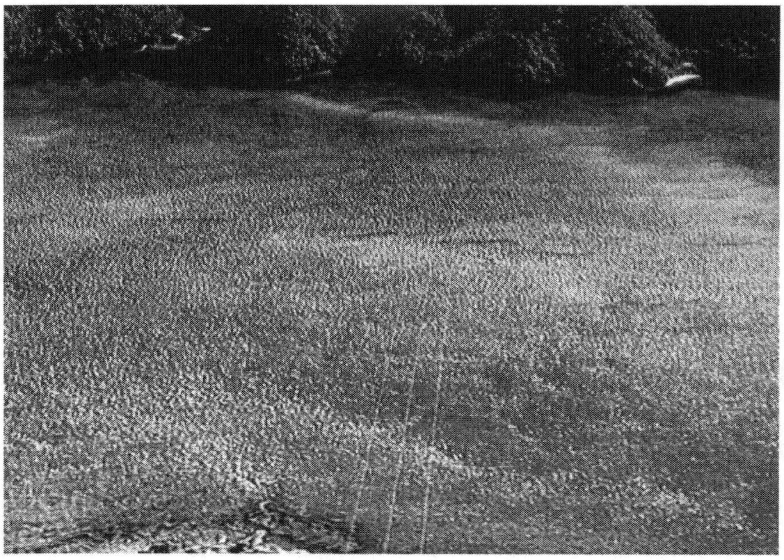

The Tory Channel cables may be visible from satellites but are invisible to pilots approaching at the same level as the wires. (Google Earth)

Investigations became protracted and the accident report was not released until February 1988. The Teledyne Continental IO-520-F engine had been installed in 1981 and was last overhauled in the United States prior to the aircraft being exported to New Zealand in 1984. The logbooks showed that on at least two occasions since overhaul, parts had had to be replaced and on one occasion rough running had necessitated an immediate return to land where a broken cylinder had to be removed. Extensive enquiries were made of the engine manufacturers and also of the facility that had carried out the last overhaul. While it was not mandatory to replace certain parts in the United States, it was a requirement in New Zealand, and it was found that certain components should have been replaced before the engine entered air transport work in New Zealand. Inconsistencies were found in the engine log book entries: one New Zealand engineer had written 'connecting rod bolt (renewed) at overhaul' when it was clearly impossible to make such a statement. The surveyor who endorsed this log entry came in for heavy criticism when the accident report was finally released.

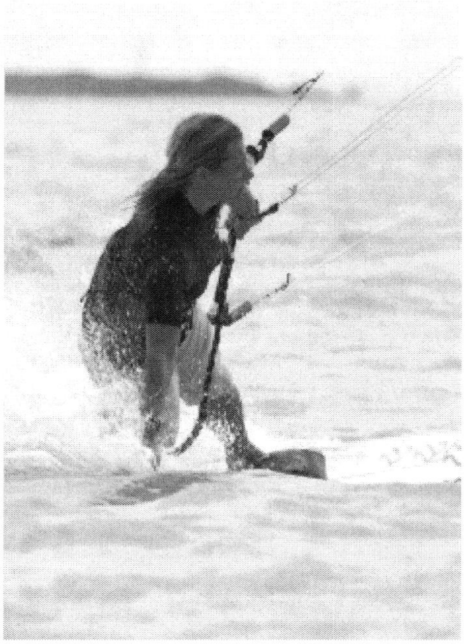

Cindy Mosey, the only survivor of the 1985 Tory Channel air crash. She later became world kite-surfing champion in 2006, 2007 and 2008. (Cindy Mosey)

The actions of the 44-year-old pilot, Winston Cunliffe, initially RNZAF-trained and a highly ranked airline captain with 10,781 hours experience, were not faulted.

Following the Erebus disaster in 1979, the aviation fraternity became more familiar with terms such as ocular illusion, sector whiteout, slant visibility, distance perception, and the human factors that come into play when a VFR pilot is confronted with difficult weather conditions. But the pilot of a Soundsair Cessna Caravan flight from Wellington to Picton on 29 January 1996 entered an area of sector whiteout with fatal consequences for his six passengers. The aircraft departed Wellington at 4.10p.m. to fly VFR to the Picton airstrip at Koromiko. The usual procedure was to fly to the northern end of Cloudy Bay at Rarangi, turn right into the Tuamarina valley and follow the valley for about three miles to the airstrip, a flight the pilot had conducted hundreds of times before without incident.

In Cloudy Bay an onshore breeze gave rise to misty fog at low level, overcast cloud above, with clear air between the two layers of cloud. Flying between the two layers, it was most likely still possible to fly by Visual Flight Rules. The pilot of a Cessna 172 heading for D'Urville Island at 4.20p.m., intending to transit through the same Tuamarina valley, found it blocked with fog. As he diverted to the Okaramio valley further to the west, he heard the Caravan give his position 'at Rununder Point' but heard nothing more. At 4.27p.m., with the slopes of Mt Robertson obscured by fog, the Cessna Caravan approached through an area of almost zero visibility and when the trees suddenly came into the pilot's view, he attempted a steep climbing turn but was unable to avoid crashing into the trees.

As the only survivor, the pilot was able to give evidence in the ensuing investigation, where he was found culpable for the accident. He later pleaded guilty to a charge of manslaughter and was sentenced. Some commentators were sympathetic to the pilot's position and wrote in some detail about the technical issues, explaining how easy it was for a VFR pilot to fall into such a trap. It was pointed out that when flying between two layers of cloud a false horizon can appear due to another type of visual illusion known as the Mach effect. While the regulations mandate minimum conditions for VFR flight, in reality, weather conditions can change with deceptive speed to the point where, technically, the flight should be discontinued to avoid breaching those regulations. While this may sound easy enough to comply with, in practice – and particularly over water or inhospitable terrain – it is sometimes not possible to divert from an existing flight path without actually increasing the level of danger.

He later pleaded guilty to a charge of manslaughter and was sentenced.

It is said that with more experience a pilot is able to judge well ahead to determine the point to turn away safely from developing danger ahead. But the difficulties are magnified and compounded when flights are scheduled to depart and arrive at fixed times and these pressures are placed on the flight crew.

In high winds the Marlborough Sounds can be one of the most challenging aviation environments on the planet, with severe turbulence and sudden downdraughts making control of a light aircraft difficult even for the most experienced of pilots. By a strange coincidence, all three of these tragedies occurred within a radius of about eight kilometres, yet there were no high winds or challenging turbulence in any of them. The common cause in each case was the slip of a human hand.

27

SHE'LL BE RIGHT

The Cave Creek platform collapse 1995

On a chilly clear autumn morning in April 1995, two jumbo vans from Tai Poutini Polytechnic wended their way around Greymouth uplifting 17 warmly kitted-out students for a planned field trip to visit various geological features in Paparoa Forest Park, 18 kilometres north of the town. A similar-sized group from the same outdoor recreation course had taken the trip the day before, enthusing them with anticipation of a relaxing day in the bush.

Without exception the students were enjoying the course, bonded together through a love of the wild West Coast. Despite the presence of many West Coast pubs, these students were less inclined to embark on pub crawls than their Dunedin counterparts might have been, but were more likely to be found enjoying fish and chips on Cobden beach with the sun going down. Adventure tourism was on the rise, opening an array of job opportunities throughout New Zealand and overseas. The future was bright and everyone was excited.

When in the 1980s tertiary education in New Zealand received a makeover, polytechnics descended on small towns with a growing variety of educational courses. A few short years before, school leavers would slot into any job they could find, perhaps study part-time at a night class or by correspondence, perhaps take an apprenticeship. Those with a studious bent were firmly directed to a university in one of the main centres. When Tai Poutini Polytechnic in Greymouth offered a full-time outdoor recreation course, it became a magnet for students all around New Zealand. Enrolments for 1995 came from as far north as Maungaturoto and as far south as Invercargill.

The vans stopped at Punakaiki to pick up Shirley Slatter, information manager of the Department of Conservation (DOC) centre, then proceeded to the end of Bullock Creek Road. Here they were joined by Stephen O'Dea, manager of the Punakaiki visitor centre, and John Skilton of Tai Poutini Polytechnic. Shirley led the students through a lecture and discussion on the geological features of the area, pointing out where Bullock Creek entered an underground course through a submergence known as Taurus Major, to emerge at the Cave Creek resurgence some distance away. The vehicles took them to the start of a track leading to the resurgence. The group walked for about half an hour through a bush track to a viewing platform overlooking the point where Cave Creek joins the Pororari River. Towards the end of this walk, John and Shirley waited for three slower members of the group, one of whom, Leanne Wheeler, was hampered with a sore knee.

Stephen O'Dea led the students in single file on to the viewing platform, which was soon bearing the full weight of eighteen people. On the previous day's visit Shirley Slatter had noticed some movement in the platform and mentioned it to Stephen O'Dea. During the bush walk in, she suggested he check out any flexing on the structure. One or two students looked over the edge and recoiled at the sheer drop to the rocks 120 feet below. Some of the students began shaking the platform, which resonated into a rocking motion that was noticed by others in the group. Suddenly the structure started to slope downwards at an increasingly sharp angle, then it separated completely from its supports, sending all 18 on the platform in free fall all the way to the rocky ground below. Eleven of them were killed outright, two were seriously injured, and another two died before help arrived.

The small group at the top could hear shouts from below and someone calling out for help. Mark Traynor was detailed to go back to raise the alarm while the remainder of the group began to descend to render first aid to those below. Shirley started writing instructions for Mark to make a call using a radio-telephone in one of the vehicles, then realised it would be too complicated a task, so both Mark and Shirley ran back to the vehicles, only to find that the keys needed to switch on the radios were in Stephen

O'Dea's pocket. Mark Traynor then began running the seven kilometres back to Punakaiki to raise the alarm.

One or two students looked over the edge and recoiled at the sheer drop to the rocks 120 feet below.

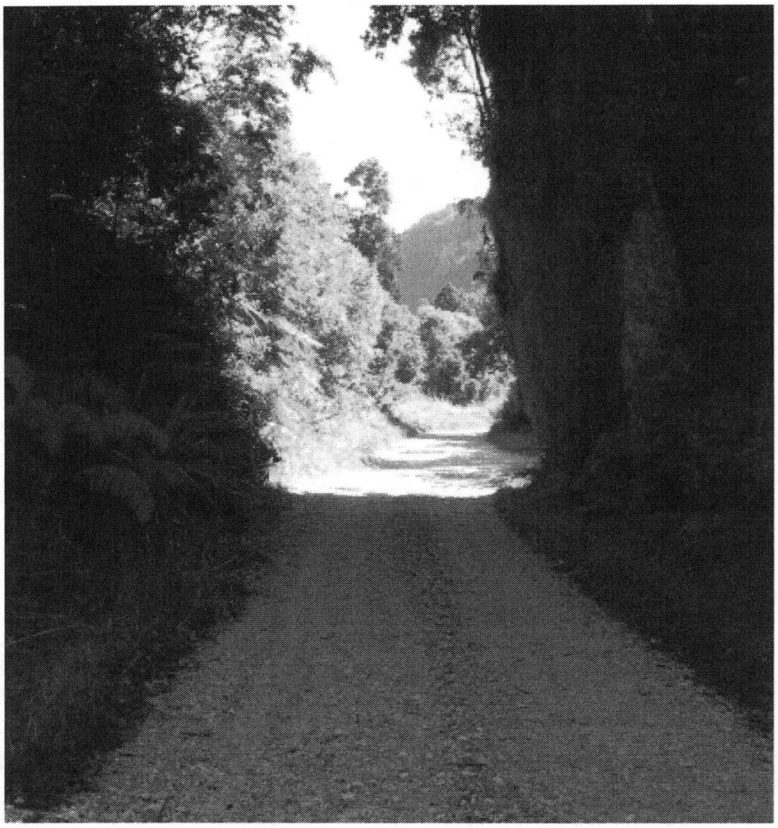

Miles from anywhere. Mark Traynor dashed 7 kilometres along Bullock Creek Road to raise the alarm following the Cave Creek platform collapse. (Russell Young)

While Shirley was returning to the accident site she encountered two cyclists on the road, one of whom was deemed fit enough to pursue Mark to allow him use of his bicycle. Before sending him on his way,

Shirley wrote out more instructions to be given to Mark to relay to the police. When the cyclist caught up with Mark he was able to continue the journey by bicycle and reached a farm house 1 km north of Punakaiki belonging to Jack Forrest. Owing to his state of exhaustion, Mark was unable to read the full list of instructions, so Mr Forrest completed the 111 call, which was made to Greymouth Police Station at 12.16p.m.

Meanwhile John Skilton, Leanne Wheeler and Darren Gamble were confronting the tangled mass of bodies at the foot of the cliff. To lessen the impact of shock, John Skilton warned the students, as best he could, of what they were likely to face. Two of the students, Stacy Mitchell and Scott Murray, were conscious and after being freed, able to move about, and a third, Carolyn Smith, was conscious but her leg badly broken. When the remaining bodies were checked for breathing and pulse, a further three, Sam Lucas, Kit Pawsey and Stephen Hannen were found to be still alive, although Kit was unconscious and Stephen showed signs of serious spinal injuries. While they were helping move the survivors into the recovery position, they found that Kit Pawsey had died. After carefully checking all the bodies, it was clear to the rescuers that the others were dead.

When Shirley Slatter returned, she searched for some time for keys to the vehicles to enable radio calls, the first being put out by 12.50p.m. By this time, in response to the 111 call, the first helicopter was on its way to the scene. This was locally operated by Chris Cowan of Coastwide Helicopters, who as a matter of course received the first call for any rescue assistance on the West Coast. The magnitude of the disaster had been well transmitted and both the Westpac Rescue helicopter and an RNZAF Iriquois were on their way from Christchurch. Shortly after the first patient had been lifted out by Chris Cowan, the rescue party noticed that Scott Murray had stopped breathing, and despite the efforts of Shirley Slatter, John Skilton and Constable Joyce (who had just arrived) to keep him alive, it became obvious after about 15 minutes that they were not successful and CPR was stopped. During this period, Carolyn Smith was also evacuated, Stephen Hannen was winched to the Westpac helicopter and Stacy Mitchell was lifted out by the Iriquois.

By about 2p.m. the police, four ambulances, two fire engines, a rescue tender and three helicopters were on site, despite the leading ambulance becoming stalled in a flooded ford on Bullock Creek Road and blocking all access for several chaotic minutes. By this time, Shirley Slatter, Darren Gamble, Leanne Wheeler and John Skilton were able to leave matters to the growing team of police, emergency and ambulance workers whose main task now was attending to the removal of bodies. As news of the disaster spread nationwide, the expected media contingent invaded the area, resulting in the Polytechnic, the Punakaiki visitor centre, the hospital and police station being deluged with frantic calls. At 5p.m. the police telecommunications system collapsed.

Not all the families of the victims were happy with the way in which they received news of the death of their son or daughter, protocol requiring such news to be delivered in person and not by telephone. Many parents phoned in and were told nothing, or were told to go to their local police station, produce identification and make enquiries there. Messages could only be sent around the country to the various police stations through the police computer network after appropriate procedures had been carried out, which happened after 7p.m. By this time, several stations were unattended and some messages simply popped up on a screen in an empty room. However, most families were properly notified by a police officer between 7.45p.m. and 10.45p.m. One family in Canada received a visit at 5.45a.m. local time (12.45a.m. NZT).

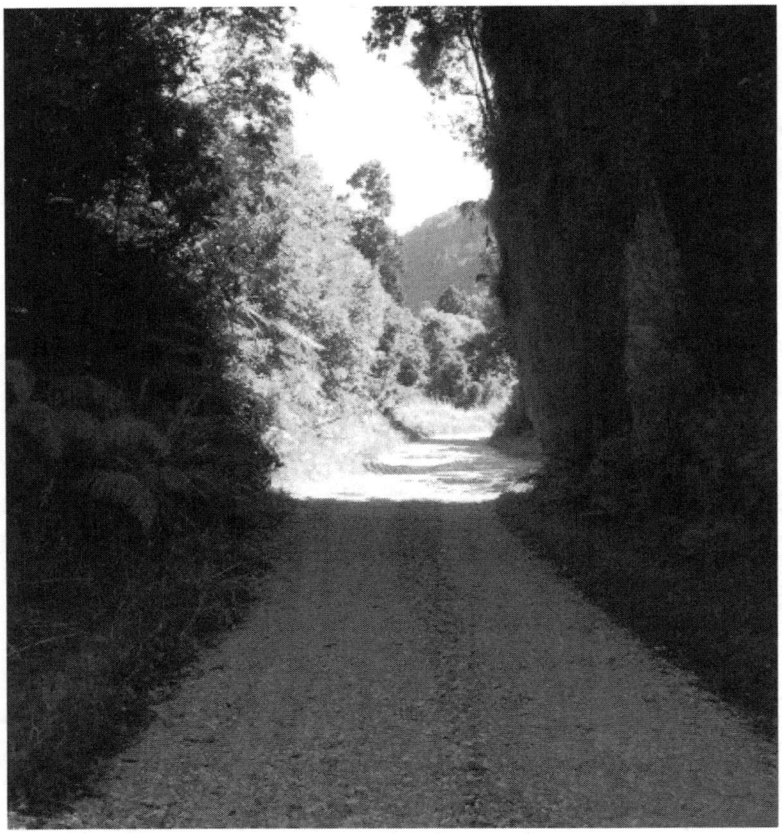

A helicopter hovers to evacuate victims of the Cave Creek disaster. (Fairfax New Zealand)

The grief of many families turned to anger when the Commission of Enquiry began its hearing a few weeks later, uncovering unbelievable negligence on an unprecedented scale.

The Department of Conservation was set up out of a major restructure of many government departments in 1987. The days of a safe government job for life vanished overnight. Many jobs were restructured into a format that made them accountable and where possible any user of government services was to be charged some sort of fee. Various functions previously carried out by the Lands and Survey, NZ Forest Service, NZ Wildlife Service and the Archaeology Section of Internal Affairs were combined to create the new department. Every government department was busy doing strategic plans. The Commission of Enquiry, and many critics of the new regime, considered that from the outset the department was seriously underfunded for the tasks it was supposed to carry out. As a result, many staff members were working long hours and were frustrated at every turn by lack of funding for essential materials. Thus it was found that the cost of proper engineering reports for projects such as the Cave Creek platform would have been simply impossible to contemplate.

Throughout the department, in keeping with its origins and heritage, Kiwi ingenuity became a recognised substitute for proper building and engineering qualifications. Thus the design plans for the Cave Creek platform were prepared by a former A-grade mechanic. The plans were submitted for approval to the Northern Operations Manager based at Hokitika, Kevin Wilde, on 4 November 1992 and approved within 24 hours. The platform was then assembled at Punakaiki and lifted by helicopter to the Cave Creek site in December 1992, where it remained until April 1993 when a DOC work party of four set about installing it with hammer and nails.

The ad hoc foreman was a former freezing worker, fencing contractor and general hand, assisted by Kevin Wilde and two others. The motor mechanic's plans were neither taken to the site nor followed, and the work party was later heavily lambasted for this. Missing from the installation was a steel bar to connect with bolts to a Kiwi-ingenuity-style counterweight. Engineering opinion produced during the enquiry later indicated that, while the plans were substandard in many respects, a properly connected counterweight would have prevented collapse.

On several occasions following installation, queries were raised about a building permit and engineering approval, but it was not until September 1994 that proactive steps were made to obtain a building permit. On closer inspection by personnel within the department, it was found the structure differed from the plans. As a German exchange student working with DOC on a three-month volunteer basis had some draughting experience, she was asked to produce some drawings, but accurate plans were impossible without dismantling the structure, so the well-intended plans were unusable. In October 1994 the department was flatly informed by Buller District Council that building permits could not be issued retrospectively. Thus no permit was obtained.

Missing from the installation was a steel bar to connect with bolts to a Kiwi-ingenuity-style counterweight.

The plight of the victims was taken up by an unlikely publication, the *National Business Review.* Graeme Hunt, a highly qualified and regarded journalist, produced a series of articles calling for accountability for the deaths. He then released a book in August 1996 entitled *Scandal at Cave Creek: A shocking failure of public accountability.* Words such as 'crimes', 'criminal acts', 'murder' and 'criminal manslaughter' slipped readily from his pen, and those responsible were unashamedly referred to as 'killers'. But the department and its employees were immune from prosecution under existing Acts of Parliament. A few limp resignations followed, and the government tried to make amends by paying out token recompense to the families of the victims.

But the department and its employees were immune from prosecution.

Everyone tried to move on with their lives. Most of those connected in any way with the disaster either moved away from the area or left for a different job. The Minister of Conservation resigned. Those students who survived the tragedy expressed nothing but goodwill towards the Department of Conservation. Stephen Hannen slowly recovered, but was confined for the rest of his life to a wheelchair. In later life he volunteered for a mentoring programme in New Brighton schools and became highly regarded encouraging young people with disabilities. Leanne Wheeler, Darren Gamble, Mark Traynor, John Skilton and Shirley Slatter were awarded the Queen's Service Medal in the 1997 New Year's and Queen's Birthday honours lists.

But one thing did change. Over the following ten years, departmental staff walked every metre of every track under their survey. Every DOC structure from Cape Reinga to Stewart Island was properly examined, scrutinised and categorised. Many structures were rebuilt, this time with proper engineering reports and building expertise, and funding flowed unimpeded. All DOC staff were proud of their efforts. It was as if the department had discovered a source of funds previously hidden underground.

28

SURE TO RISE

Tongariro canyoning tragedy 2008

A growing desire to reach out, touch and experience New Zealand's places of natural beauty in the great outdoors-mountain peaks, glaciers, caves, tracks, rivers, lakes and streams-saw an Outdoor Pursuits Centre established as a charitable trust at Tongariro in the central North Island in 1973, with the country's most famous son, Sir Edmund Hillary, named as its patron. The centre was thus named the Sir Edmund Hillary Outdoor Pursuits Centre (OPC), but just a few short weeks after he died in January 2008, the enterprise became embroiled in a disaster that took the lives of six students and one teacher from Elim Christian College in Auckland.

Jodie Sullivan, 26, joined the instructing staff at OPC in January 2008. She was instantly well liked and widely regarded as outstanding, with people saying she had the 'X factor'. She had gained a Bachelor of Physical Education degree from the University of Otago in 2006, followed by some relevant adventure experience, and had completed a twelve-week training course in December 2007. Each instructor needed to be trained and signed off on applicable competencies before instructing on the various activities. Students were normally divided into groups with a ratio of ten students to one instructor to maintain a minimum standard of safety, and schools were asked to arrange grouping in advance. Forty students and two staff from Elim Christian College in Greenmount, Auckland, arrived at the centre on Sunday, 13 April 2008 to undertake a five-day standard Summer Adventure Challenge embracing two unit standards which could be applied towards a tertiary qualification. Also attending that week were groups from Melville High School and Central Hawke's Bay College, plus others attending as individuals to complete unit standards towards an instructing diploma.

Based on similar principles to the Outward Bound Trust at Anakiwa in the Marlborough Sounds, the OPC accepted enrolments from anybody willing to extend their personal boundaries, step out of their comfort zone and engage in a wide range of adventure and confidence-building activities. These were considered safe when conducted under the supervision of trained guides, but were dangerous, and often impossible, if conducted alone.

Over its first 35 years, the Hillary Outdoor Pursuit Centre conducted over 100,000 enthusiasts through its range of adventures. Courses were categorised into unit standards and marketed accordingly, with most participants in supervised groups from schools, ski clubs or other places where youth converge. Adult groups devoted to leadership development and team building also participated. The founder and first chairman was Graeme Dingle ONZM, MBE, widely respected for his mountaineering feats. The site was on Hydro Access Road 3, about 1 km off State Highway 47 linking Turangi with National Park, with accommodation, meeting and dining areas, and offices.

Three years after its inception, the first fatality occurred. In typical rainy weather a group of fourth-form girls were walking through the stream in Mangatepopo Gorge when the river began to rise. The OPC instructor with the group was helping them exit to safety one by one when one girl lost her balance, was swept away and drowned under a jumble of logs. The following year a register of accidents and incidents was initiated, which revealed later that several incidents occurred during periods when the river rose suddenly, and on more than one occasion a person had been swept away but was rescued. Numerous safety policies and procedures were documented, kept under constant review and subject to triennial audit.

There was typically a staff of around 24, including 18 instructors, with nine normally in attendance. They were highly qualified, and the CEO had a doctorate degree. However, knowledge and experience arising from previous accidents tended to dissipate due to a relatively high turnover of instructing staff. Management staff kept a growing library of data devoted to safety, monitoring of competencies, quality management, risk analysis and management, and a log of reported incidents, each with a recommendation to prevent a recurrence. The paper trail was robust.

Risk was seen as part and parcel of adventurous activity.

Parents of students sent to the Summer Adventure Challenge were advised that, depending on the season, activities would include kayaking, canoeing, tubing, rock climbing, snow and ice climbing, caving, tramping, skiing, gorge walking, camping and confidence courses. They were advised that all the activities, while supervised by highly skilled instructors, did contain some element of risk, but were assured the OPC had 'an enviable safety record'. Risk was seen as part and parcel of adventurous activity. Parents were reminded that Sir Edmund Hillary had been exposed to massive risks in conquering Everest, a mountain that had claimed so many lives in attempts on its summit that for many years it was deemed impossible to climb.

A number of students from the Elim College contingent had disabilities, but the staff were convinced the adventure course would be very good for them. One, Tom Tsu, had cerebral palsy and was accompanied at all times by a teacher, Tony McClean. Two others had swimming limitations and another, Ashley Smith, was severely short-sighted. Organisation of a normal day's activity was left to the discretion of the instructors, one of the options being a traverse through the Mangatepopo Gorge about 1 km from the Centre itself.

Two activities were normally available: the upstream course, where the party waded upstream through the river, and the downstream course, which involved floating or swimming downstream in the direction of the current. Once the gorge was entered on the downstream course, the group was more or less committed to complete the traverse as there were only two exit points, but these required abseiling to climb out and were subject to a separate level of instructor competence. After meeting her group of ten students and one teacher in the morning of 15 April 2008, Jodie Sullivan outlined the day's activities, which included a gorge trip in the afternoon.

An integral part of all safety arrangements was first to check the weather forecast, which, under a standing arrangement with MetService, was faxed to OPC at 6.45a.m. each morning. Over time, OPC found actual conditions frequently differed from those predicted by MetService, so they tended to downplay the importance of the reports. The weather report faxed to OPC on 15 April 2008 was based on observations taken at 1a.m. Part of the report read: 'Today, rain with isolated and poor visibility at times. Rain easing to showers tonight.' The word 'thunderstorms' was somehow missed from this report. The report formed part of the 7.30a.m. briefing given by OPC Operations Manager Beverley Smith and Field Manager Kerry Palmer, who had just returned from six weeks' recreational leave. They discussed the weather but did not look at the maps included with the reports.

After the briefing concluded, MetService issued a severe weather warning for the Tongariro area, but as OPC did not subscribe to this particular service, it did not receive a fax, and was later criticised for not obtaining such information from the internet.

Jodie's group spent the morning on a rope course in periods of rain, and at one stage a clap of thunder was heard. Two more experienced instructors, Peter Zimmer and Matthew Rowley, had planned gorge trips for the afternoon but decided the weather looked 'spooky' and called their trips off. Jodie had been signed off to take groups through either the downstream or the upstream course, but had not been signed off to conduct groups through the exit points. Later in the morning, Kerry Palmer visited the river to check water flow and spoke with Jodie about the afternoon gorge trip. He mentioned the possibility the river might rise, but Jodie reassured him the group would not be venturing too far into the gorge or going anywhere she would not go herself.

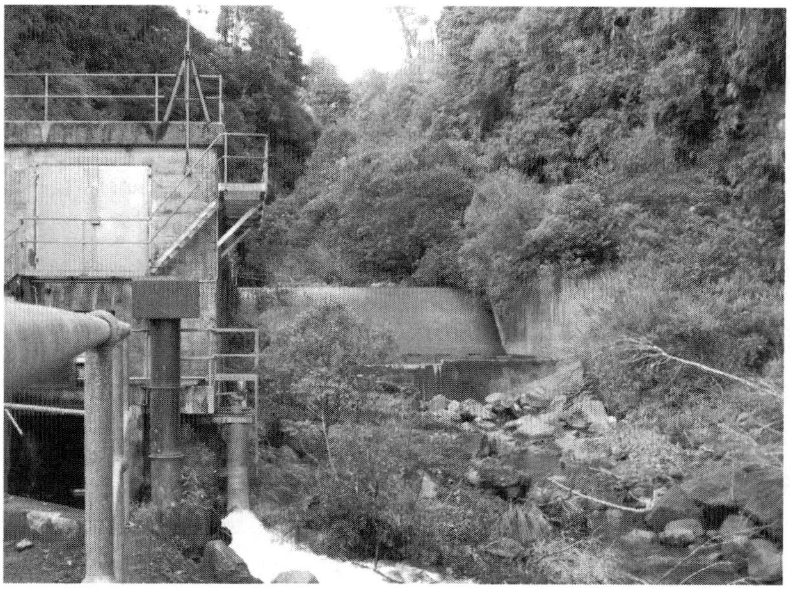

The Mangatepopo weir in normal water flow, but on 15 April 2008 these rocks lay beneath torrents of floodwater. (Russell Young)

After lunch, Jodie's group entered the gorge, walking upstream for about a third of the normal distance for an upstream course. They passed by a flat ledge but decided to retrace their steps as the stream was starting to rise, frightening some in the group. Returning by the same ledge, they found the water had risen sharply, the streambed impassable. They retreated to the safety of the ledge which was quickly invaded, forcing everyone to stand on slippery rock in water rising up to their calves, as the stream turned into an angry torrent of brown water. The noise was deafening, making it almost impossible to pass on instructions.

The group waited in vain for the river to subside, then after nearly an hour made the decision to vacate the ledge and ride the current downstream to safety. The two weakest students were linked by rope to an adult, Ashley Smith to Jodie, and Tom Hsu to his teacher, Antony McClean. The plan was for Jodie to go first and assist the others to exit a short distance down the river, out of sight around a corner, by using a 'throwbag' technique, where a rope in a bag was thrown to the person in the river enabling them to use the current to float to the bank where Jodie would pull them out.

He missed the throwbag and was washed over the weir.

Jodie and Ashley went first and pulled themselves out of the river a short distance from a weir. Anyone left in the river at that point would be cascaded over the weir onto logs and slabs of concrete. There was to be a five-minute gap between each person, to enable Jodie and Ashley to position themselves in readiness but, sooner than expected, Kish Proctor came around the corner alone, but on the wrong side of the river. He missed the throwbag and was washed over the weir, losing his helmet and boots, but was able to scramble ashore below the weir. He was followed quickly by Peter Shiih who managed to grab the rope and was successfully pulled from the river.

It was now 4.05p.m., and Jodie succeeded in making a radio call back to OPC seeking urgent assistance. At this moment Portia McPhail came around the corner, initially missed the rope, grabbed it again, was washed over the weir losing hold of the rope and was swept away. Natasha Bray came next, managed to grab the rope, lost her grip and was also swept over the weir. Floyd Fernandes and Anthony Mulder, roped together to assist the weaker swimmer, came past, missed the rope and, too far out to be grabbed to safety, were washed away. Tara Gregory followed, suffering a similar fate. Next came Sarah Brooks who missed the throwrope but managed to hold on to a wire stretching above the weir. She was washed over the weir but survived. The last pair to come down, Tom Hsu and Antony McClean, managed to grab the throwrope but the current was too strong and they were swept away together. Altogether, six students and one teacher had lost their lives in the space of ten minutes.

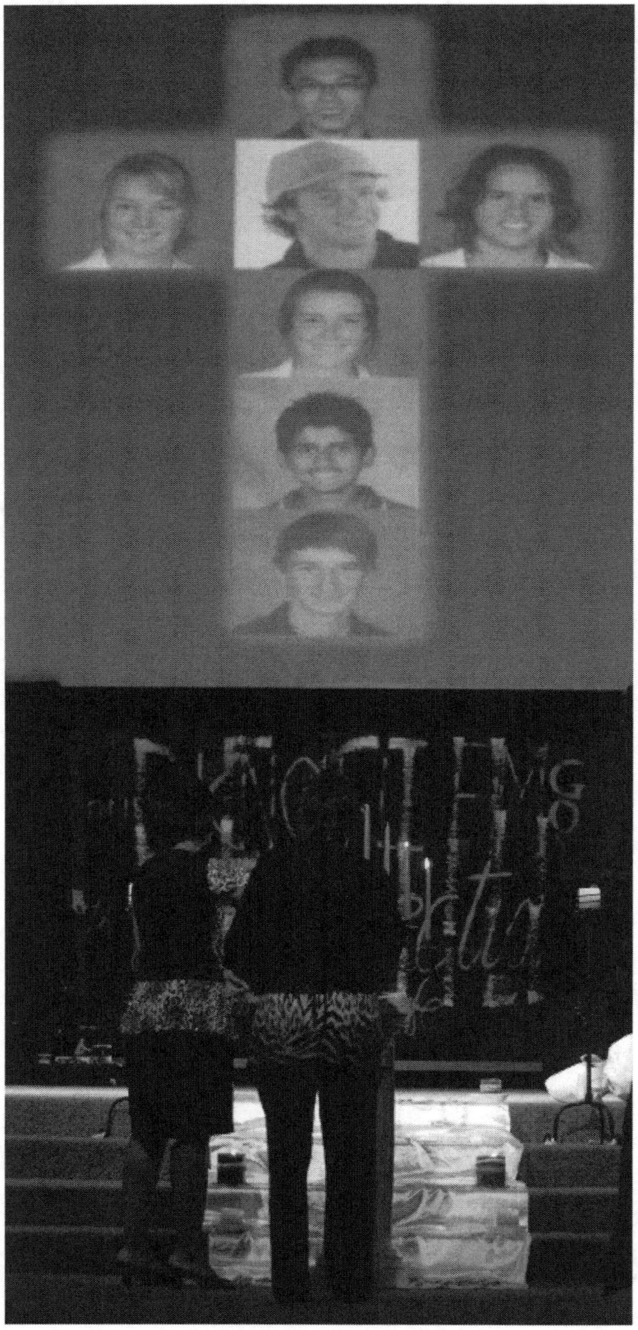

Mothers of students who died light candles at a service at Elim Christian College to mark the first anniversary of the Mangatepopo tragedy. (Richard Robinson/New Zealand Herald)

The enquiry was not completed until November 2009, and the Coroner's report signed off nearly two years after the disaster in March 2010. Some were quick to blame Jodie Sullivan, saying the group would all have survived if they had just waited on the ledge for the water to drop. That was easy to say from a desk, with access to rainfall and riverflow data, not so easy when a rising torrent was coursing over your knees and the lives of ten students and one teacher were in your hands. If they remained on the ledge and the water continued to rise, they would all be swept to certain death. The enquiry found that just as the group left the ledge, the water was actually starting to subside.

The Outdoor Pursuit Centre was quick to acknowledge blame, conceding numerous breaches of safety procedure, pleading guilty to various charges and accepting a penalty of $450,000. The CEO resigned. MetService accepted that its early forecast was, inexplicably, incomplete but pointed out that it had issued updates with appropriate warnings. Virtually all Elim College hearts reached out with compassion and forgiveness to Jodie Sullivan, who was too overcome to complete her testimony at the enquiry and declined to take part in restorative justice meetings. She stayed on at OPC for a year before departing for a job in America. In 2011 Antony McClean and Anthony Mulder were recognised with posthumous bravery awards for putting their own lives at risk in their vain attempts to save Tom Hsu and Floyd Fernandes, and the principal, Murray Burton, was awarded the New Zealand Order of Merit for his role in supporting the school and the families through the aftermath. *North and South* magazine named him New Zealander of the Year in 2008.

Most parents of Elim College students were supportive of OPC and were happy for the courses to continue, but in 2009 the college decided not to return for the immediate future. A memorial scholarship was established, and on the fifth anniversary of the disaster a dedicated climbing wall was erected at Elim College. The seven who died are remembered at the school as 'The Seven in Heaven'.

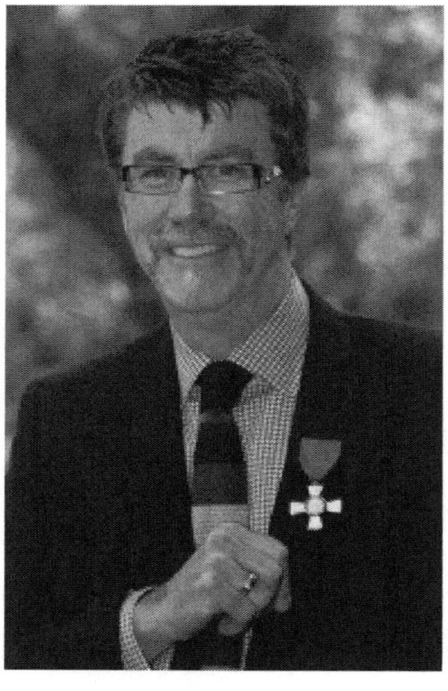

The principal of Elim College, Murray Burton, received the New Zealand Order of Merit for his handling of the Tongariro canyoning disaster. (New Zealand Herald)

29

COLD COMFORT AT THE COALFACE

The Pike River Mine explosion 2010

Go to a rugby match on the West Coast and chances are it will be raining as locals arrive in twos and threes, eventually clumping together with their umbrellas on the sideline. Sheltered from the rain, someone will be cooking sausages or whitebait fritters, stray aromas inviting a steady trickle of patronage. Talk to any Coaster there and you can have a conversation with anyone about anything at all, with ease. But after the game as you start to leave, you will find yourself looking at many retreating backs.

They say you are not usually taken up as a Coaster until you have lived on the coast yourself for a decade or two, or are part of a family dating back a few generations. Something invisible ties them together, not so much to keep others out, but to ensure that those in their midst are true to their bond. Maybe this is due to exposure to the lifelong danger of working underground, a danger accepted, shared and passed on from generation to generation. If you are just a visitor you are not likely to share the depth of their bonds, not really. The money is good, it is a hard job and, yes, there are risks which they say are just part of life. Everyone knows someone who has lost a friend killed in a mining accident.

While everyone in the industry did their best to comply with health and safety standards, and all mines installed vastly improved ventilation systems, accidents and earthfalls still occurred. The chemical equation is the same anywhere on the globe and has never changed: when a carbonaceous seam of rock is disturbed, methane gas is released. In days gone by, the foreman would carry a canary into the mine to indicate dangerous methane levels, but now there are digitally triggered warning systems and workers at all times carry a rescue kit with 30 minutes' worth of oxygen, sufficient to exit the mine in times of trouble. They say that provided safety standards are observed, someone would need to make a serious mistake to trigger an explosion.

A number of facts had become obvious to Coasters over the years, some learned the hard way at the expense of a few lives. Geological fault lines running through strata indicate unstable ground which is inherently at risk of collapse or seepage of deadly methane. The operation must be well capitalised due to the high cost of setting up. In the case of Pike River Mine, it was also widely known that the coal samples obtained from test drilling there emitted high levels of methane. If conventional machinery proved ineffective, proposed methodology using high-pressure water directed at the rock face inside the mine would produce uncontrolled levels of methane.

Despite the enormous challenges to be overcome in extracting coal through tunnelling rather than open casting, Grey District Mayor Tony Kokshoorn expended several years of high energy promoting the establishment of the Pike River Mine. The sheer size of the resource would surely become a magnet for job creation and provide a much-needed economic boost to the entire region. During the 1990s many extractive industries on the West Coast had quietly petered out, often in response to union pressure or environmental concerns, leading to the loss of hundreds of jobs and a corresponding population drop from 40,000 to 30,000. The days of mining families with son following father into a lifelong career underground faded with the closure of mines. Many people left the Coast permanently, leading to the ironic position that there were insufficient experienced miners left on the Coast to take up the jobs created at Pike River.

The company embarked on a vigorous overseas recruitment campaign which resulted in a diverse multinational workforce. Where in days gone by the workforce was heavily controlled by the unions who could enforce changes through strike action, at Pike River much of the workforce consisted of independent contractors and the power of the unions to insist on a safe working environment was dissipated. The workforce came from Great Britain, Australia, South Africa, the United States and the Pacific Islands, mixed, at Kokshoorn's insistence, with a solid representation of locals.

Pike River Coal Company (PRC) was an offshoot of New Zealand Oil and Gas (NZOG), a survivor of the 1987 sharemarket crash, with 26 years' successful trading under its belt. A massive underground seam of coking coal, believed to be New Zealand's largest, had been surveyed in the Paparoa ranges. It was estimated that production would exceed a million tonnes by the end of year three. Worldwide demand for coking coal saw the public issue of PRC shares in July 2007 heavily oversubscribed. Well before completion of access tunnels and associated infrastructure, a spike in the world price for coking coal forced the share price upwards, making it the top-performing stock on the New Zealand Stock Exchange in 2008.

But in August 2008 everyone was still waiting for the access tunnel to hole through. Then management were looking for outcomes that would see the mine 'de-risked', and market analysts debated which method might be applied to value the operation, which could possibly be sold off as a going concern once full production kicked in. The share price hit $2.45, one analyst predicting it 'could go north of $3'. The mine was officially opened in November 2008, but less than six months later the company was strapped for cash and needed to float more shares to fund infrastructure and address a raft of problems arising from an 'unexpected' rockfall. Management trod the tricky path of raising a further $45 million without revealing the full extent of their problems, thereby denting investor confidence. However, in May 2009 the share issue was again oversubscribed.

Management became niggly, arguments broke out, safety issues were neglected.

Pike River Mine stumbled along, producing a small fraction of budgeted output. A number of key personnel lost belief in the project and resigned, their replacements staying in the job only a short time before they, too, resigned. Management became niggly, arguments broke out, safety issues were neglected. With production lagging well behind schedule, staff were offered huge bonuses to press for higher levels of extraction. Saturations of methane triggered off alarms, which were deactivated so that everyone could carry on rather than addressing the problem. At a staff barbecue in 2010, a group of workers resolved that they needed to do something to shut the mine down, the general consensus being 'she's going to blow'. On 19 November 2010, as so many had predicted, the mine did explode. Out of 31 workers and contractors present in the mine, only two survived.

At 3.44p.m. the lights flickered in one of the offices and alarms in the control room were activated. Daniel Duggan was in sole charge of the surface control room when he suddenly lost contact during a conversation with a work party deep in the mine, the alarms signalling severed communication lines. Daniel Duggan passed his concerns on to the mine manager and shortly thereafter Mattheus Strydom, a contract electrician with 28 years' mining experience, entered the mine on a transport device known as a driftrunner but without a self-rescue pack. He had gone about 1500 metres when he saw a light ahead, which on closer inspection proved to be stationary with a body lying nearby. His breathing suddenly became more difficult, then the motor on his device began to falter, but he was able to run it backwards downhill, restart the motor and exit the mine with all speed.

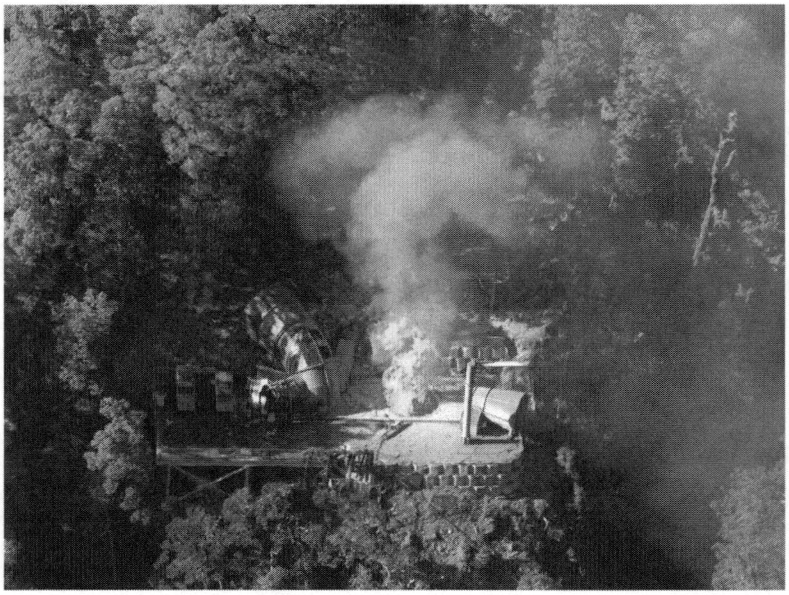

No hope of survival. Flames escape the sole ventilation shaft at Pike River Mine. (New Zealand Herald)

Elsewhere in the mine, Daniel Rockhouse was refuelling his drift-runner when he saw a white flash and was felled by a blast which knocked him unconscious. Recovering, but in extreme discomfort, he was able to find his way to a fresh air source and began to stagger towards the exit. On his way he encountered another driftrunner, with Russell Smith unconscious nearby. Daniel was able to drag Russell to what he thought was an air vent, but found it had been decommissioned. Eventually they were both able to stagger 1500 metres through the tunnels, collapsing several times, before finally reaching fresh air outside the mine. Daniel was later the reluctant recipient of a bravery award for his determination in saving Russell Smith. What he did not realise at the time was that he had lost a brother in the explosion.

Rescue crews, fire engines, ambulances and helicopters sped to the scene, to be joined at the mine entrance by many off-shift workers who quickly got word that something terrible had happened. They were all denied access – somebody might get hurt in any rescue attempt. In the clamour at the mine entrance, frustration boiled over. Then another explosion was heard and there were rumours that a gang of off-shift workers had rushed in against all warnings to attempt rescue. This rumour proved to be untrue. Later, however, at least two rescuers quit the Fire Service altogether in protest. They had been prepared to take whatever risk to rescue their mates, but had been denied.

The families of the men below were devastated when their loved ones did not come out of the mine. While exact details of the situation underground were not known, news was imparted to the families in clumsy fashion, and all were led to believe that the men could be quietly clustered around a fresh-air vent awaiting rescue. Anna Osborne, whose husband Milton had not come home at the end of the day, led a four-day vigil in the management offices, refusing to leave until appropriate action was taken to bring her husband out. But on the fifth day, counselled by Tony Kokshoorn and relenting to pleas from her two children, she went back home.

A second explosion sent fire ripping through the mine.

The police took control of the situation but could offer nothing, merely reaffirming that it would be suicidal to enter the mine to attempt rescue. Air samples had been checked, confirming the presence of explosive gas. With everyone waiting, a robot was flown in, travelled a short distance into the mine before breaking down. After five agonising days of expectation, all doubt was removed when a second explosion sent fire ripping through the mine, followed by two further explosions.

The families' plight was taken up by Bernie Monk, father of 23-year-old Michael, who was killed in the mine. A popular Paroa publican and former long-standing captain of Blaketown rugby club and West Coast provincial rugby teams, his name for many years more commonly appeared in the *New Zealand*

Rugby Almanack than in the national news. As spokesman for the families he suddenly became a national identity, news broadcasts picturing him next to a poignant photo of his son. Some months later Bernie's oldest son Alan made the West Coast Heartland rugby team, bringing a smile back to his face.

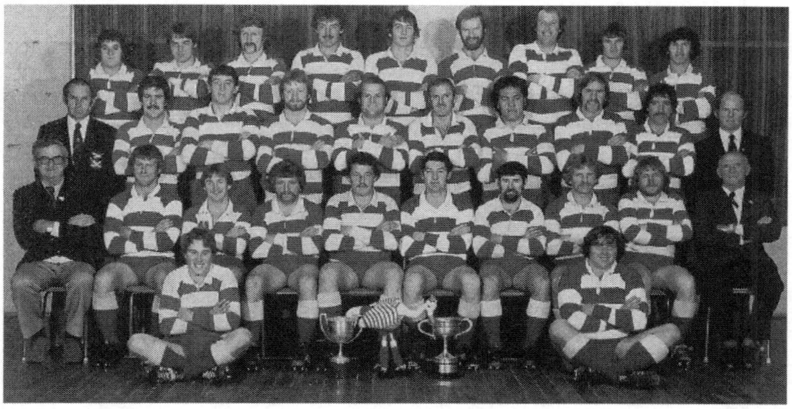

Bernie Monk (seated, fifth from left) was captain of the West Coast rugby team in 1980. (Bernie Monk)

The last voice heard from deep inside the mine before the explosion occurred belonged to a 25-year-old Scot named Joseph Campbell who, since leaving his home town of St Andrews in 2006, had worked in a variety of jobs in Australia before coming to New Zealand and scoring a job at Pike River. He was best man at the wedding of his mate Daniel Rockhouse, and had been planning to return to Australia with his girlfriend and her young daughter and get married there, his parents having already booked their fares. Daniel himself returned to work in Australian mines after the disaster.

Milton Osborne, a contractor at the mine, was serving his second term as a Grey District Councillor and left behind a wife and two children aged 11 and 13. West Coast National MP Chris Auchinvole recalled Osborne as a 'great guy' who gave good advice during the election campaign. If things got a bit rough he would tap Auchinvole on the shoulder and say, 'Chris, mate. You just stay lovely, that's how they want you. I'll do the nasty bits.'

Having just celebrated his 17th birthday, he was dead before 4p.m. the next day.

A 25-year-old drilling supervisor, Joshua Ufer from Queensland, was engaged to Rachelle Weaver, who was expecting the couple's first baby in May. Friends recalled him as a determined and hard worker who would 'punch through rock' to get out. If anyone could get out, they said, it would be him. His parents Joanne and Karl had flown to New Zealand from Australia and China. Tragically, the youngest worker, Joseph Dunbar, was due to begin work the following Monday but was so keen he was allowed to start three days early. Having just celebrated his 17th birthday, he was dead before 4p.m. the next day.

In the following days and weeks as the dust began to settle, everybody on the West Coast grieved and steps were taken to set up a Commission of Enquiry. Tony Kokshoorn became an instant media celebrity and CEO Peter Whittall's face appeared regularly on everybody's television screen throughout the enquiry.

Finally, on 30 October 2012, the 439-page report was finally signed off. Within minutes of its release, the Minister of Labour, Kate Wilkinson, resigned. They said it was the only honourable thing to do, as the enquiry found the mine inspections wanting in that they had completely failed to protect 29 innocent lives.

The mining inspectorate system had undergone considerable restructuring, ironically reducing its effectiveness. The 'old' system had seen the Chief Inspector of Mines, against considerable protest, force the closure of a Huntly mine in 1992, saving many lives, as three days later that mine had burst into flames. Pike River Coal had been left to implement its own systems which were subject to ineffectual review. Following the Pike River disaster, the inspectorate was beefed up with the establishment of a High Hazards Unit, which shut down areas of the adjacent Spring Creek Mine a few months later. But Coasters remain sceptical.

Immediately after the disaster the company was de-listed and placed in receivership. The mine remained shut permanently, with explosions and fire ripping through the tunnels at random intervals. It was never possible to retrieve the bodies in such conditions. With everybody focused on the Commission of Enquiry, the mine was quietly sold off for $32.5m to Solid Energy, realising $7.5m in cash, with the remaining $25m to be paid in instalments proportional to the actual extraction of coal.

But everyone on the Coast knew there was never any intention to extract coal: Solid Energy could recoup its $7.5m by simply selling off the infrastructure. In October 2012 a contracting company, Valley Longwall, was fined $46,800 for various safety breaches, and in June 2013 a fine of $760,000 was imposed on Pike River Coal. The receivers could only add this to the long list of unsecured creditors. As original promoter, NZOG provided $52m through a mix of secured and unsecured loans, enabling the receivership process to continue.

With everyone baying for recompense, a faltering attempt was made to prosecute Peter Whittall, who had been involved from the inception of Pike Rive Mine but had been CEO for less than two months at the time of the disaster. His immediate predecessor, Gordon Ward, had returned to Australia a few weeks before the explosion and could not be forced to return to appear before the commission. In December 2013 the charges against Whittall were dropped, just as $3.41m in cash was conjured up for the families of the victims. In December 2014 the receivers held $17m cash to meet liabilities in excess of $65m. The equation could only change if Solid Energy reopened the mine to extract more coal, which Coasters tell you will never happen in a million years.

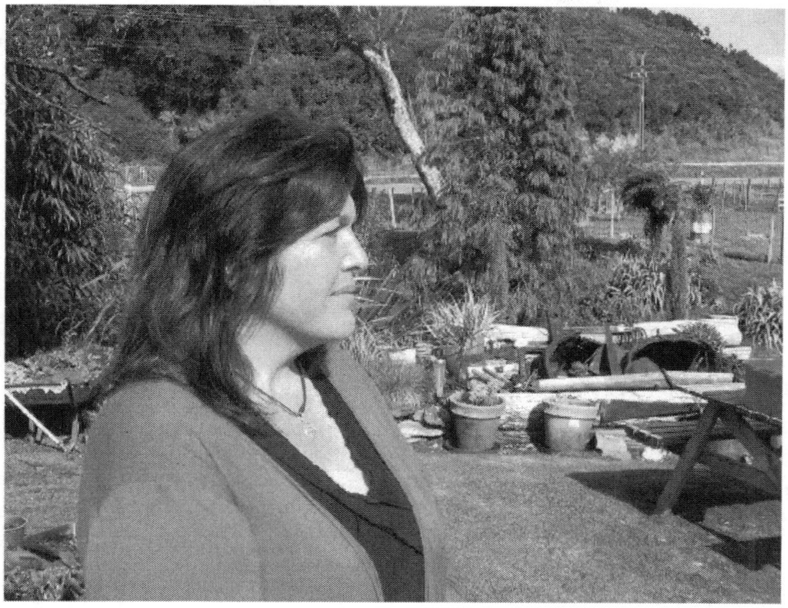

Having lost her husband at Pike River Mine in 2010, Anna Osborne in 2015 had still not held his funeral. (Russell Young)

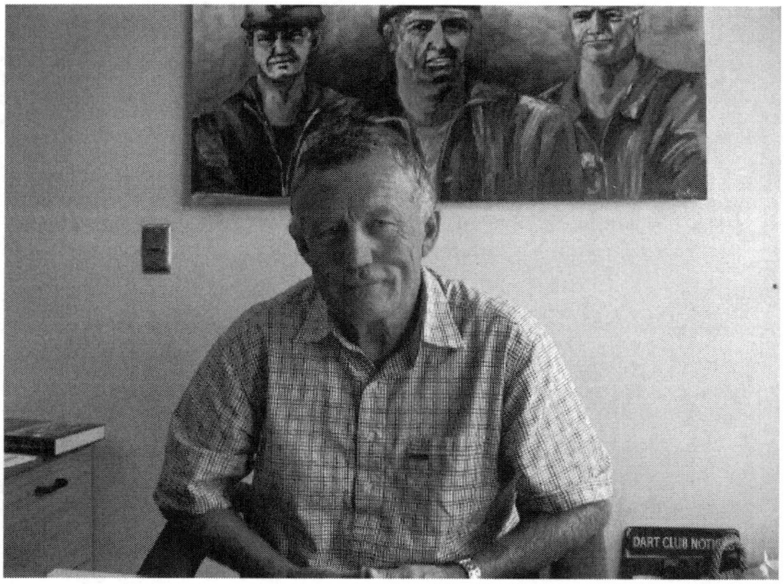

Grey District Mayor Tony Kokshoorn was automatically drawn to support Pike River Mine with its promise of economic benefit to Coasters. (Russell Young)

As an approaching election reapplied heat to the issue, the Leader of the Opposition announced he would do everything that the present government had not done. A loose promise by the Prime Minister that the government would ensure recovery of the bodies backfired, with billboards and bitter graffiti springing up in response. But by February 2015 tensions were starting to subside, bitterness slowly merging into a mood of sombre acceptance. With the mine dormant, moves were afoot to construct a memorial walkway through the area, focusing on a prime West Coast asset – its scenery.

Tony Kokshoorn summed up the tragedy of Pike River Mine in February 2015 when he said: 'The fuse of this disaster was lit when independent coal mine check inspectors ceased in the 1990s. Greed, pressure and complacency by the Pike River Coal directors and management made the explosion inevitable. May the 29 rest in peace.'

30

ON SHAKY GROUND

The Christchurch earthquake 2011

On the morning of 4 September 2010, an earthquake measuring 7.1 on the Richter scale struck the Canterbury area. There was considerable damage and if an earthquake could crack walls of buildings and leave fissures across paddocks, there were fears that human casualties would be the ultimate outcome.

New Zealanders and Cantabrians felt privileged when it was declared that no one had died in the September 2010 quake. Initially there was talk of a man with a heart condition succumbing to the tremors, but later his demise could not be attributed to the quake with certainty. Many considered Christchurch to be the lucky city and Canterbury the lucky province. That's why, some time later, when a youthful bank worker in Auckland, having picked up something on the radio during his lunch break, yelled 'there's been an earthquake in Christchurch,' most considered him a bit behind the times. Almost six months in fact, for the Christchurch earthquake had struck back in September 2010. And it was now 22 February 2011.

But this was another one. Another earthquake. Tremendous destruction of the heart of Christchurch was immediately apparent. There would be deaths this time. Christchurch was not the lucky city after all.

The February 2011 earthquake that struck Christchurch was unusual. It killed 185 people and injured several thousand, yet was not as powerful as the earlier 7.1 quake on 4 September 2010 that spared all. The fact that February's quake occurred on a fault line, was near the surface and struck close to the heart of the city made it inevitable that it would leave a greater mark than the earlier shake.

This was the earthquake that experts had spoken about over the years, predicting that one day a major quake would strike close to the surface in a highly populated area. As an earthquake-prone country, New Zealand had experienced many large quakes but they had either been deeper or in areas of a thinly populated land where death and destruction were limited, if they occurred at all.

In the February quake in Christchurch the earth movements were severe. People experienced vertical as well as horizontal motion. The nature of the bedrock led to very strong groundswells. Although it registered just 6.3 on the Richter scale, ground movements in the central business district and other city areas were three to four times more violent than those generated by the earlier quake.

The epicentre of the earthquake was little more than 10 km south-east of the CBD, near the port of Lyttelton. Because of its location and shallow depth, it was always going to be destructive. The fact that the quake struck in the lunch-hour meant that many people were on the streets. An hour earlier and many of these victims would have been off the streets and, if their places of work had withstood the quake, relatively safe. It was purely random. Some were lucky and survived. Others died.

The fact that the quake struck in the lunch-hour meant that many people were on the streets.

Falling bricks and masonry in Manchester Street and Cashel Mall killed eleven people and injured many more. These were the areas where uninjured survivors were seen to spring into action first. Despite the nerve-wracking aftershocks and the danger of further collapses, many citizens began searching for victims or, if they found people with injuries, did their best to comfort them or lift them clear of the rubble. The dead were covered with blankets or tarpaulins.

It was said that the February quake often completed the job started by the September one, in that many already stricken buildings were destroyed completely by the jarring ground movements of the later quake. Older brick-and-mortar buildings, of which Christchurch had many, were especially prone to the double-whammy effects of the two quakes.

Two city buses were crushed by the collapsing walls of buildings. Six people died and several were badly injured. Further afield in the seaside suburbs of Sumner and Redcliffs, both with ocean views and a backdrop of steep hills, the quake set boulders and rocks falling towards houses and a further five people were killed by rock falls.

The most significant loss of life occurred in the central city when the Canterbury Television and Pyne Gould Corporation buildings collapsed. The former was completely destroyed, with only the lift shaft remaining upright. The floors in the building pancaked and then a fire started, adding to the plight of rescuers and trapped victims. Eventually the CTV site accounted for 115 deaths, such was its devastation, and later enquiries into the building's stability found it to have had major structural flaws. Eighteen people in the Pyne Gould Corporation building lost their lives.

Heritage buildings were badly damaged and the Anglican Christchurch Cathedral lost its spire and suffered other serious structural damage. At first it was thought that over 20 people had been struck by the cathedral collapse, but later searches proved this not to be the case. The Catholic Cathedral of the Blessed Sacrament was also damaged, along with the Provincial Council Chambers and Lyttelton's old Timeball Station. Further out in the suburbs, a church collapsed and this time there were casualties: three organ-builders died while working on the church organ.

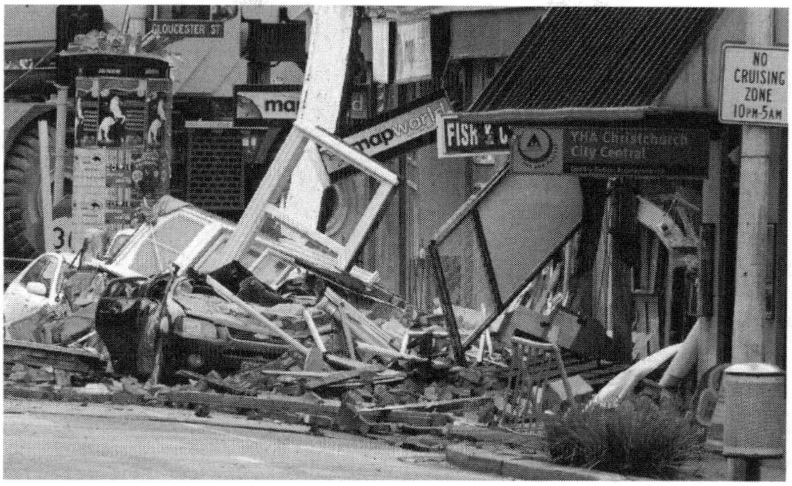

It was a busy weekday when shops in the central city resembled war zones. [Otago Daily Times]

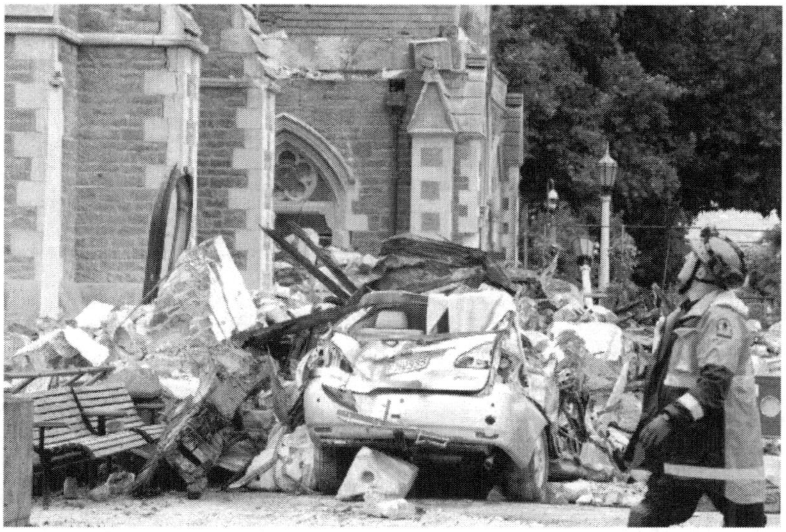

The iconic cathedral became a major casualty of the quake. It remains in limbo. (Otago Daily Times)

It was estimated that over a quarter of the buildings in the CBD were demolished in the quake. Symbolically the city's tallest building, the Hotel Grand Chancellor, was badly damaged although it was still standing.

However, it had been weakened and ended up tilting so dangerously that it was eventually demolished.

Most of New Zealand's serious disasters of the modern era have occurred in remote locations, away from the public gaze. The Tangiwai rail disaster played out its lethal course in an isolated area of the central North Island, and famously the Erebus plane crash in Antarctica occurred as far away as it is possible to get. That's why the Christchurch earthquake has left an indelible imprint on the minds of many New Zealanders who followed it closely on television and in the media in general. Not only did it occur in recent memory, but thousands of New Zealanders were able to witness the destruction and mayhem on TV.

After the initial panic and desire to get clear of falling buildings, many people wandered around in a state of shock, coming to terms with the uprooting of their city. Many had superficial injuries, others were covered in dust. One stark image showed a woman sitting on a lump of masonry with blood trickling down one cheek from a head wound and tears trickling down the other. Another showed teenagers sitting comforting one another across the road from a ruined building, waiting for word on their mother who had been working inside it.

The quake brought out the best in many. Complete strangers comforted one another. The slightly injured provided first aid for the more seriously injured. And there were cases of citizens with multiple injuries actually supporting those who were better off than them.

Then there were the heroic stories of rescue. How people caught up in the event saved lives simply because it was the thing to do. Before the official rescue teams were assembled, rank amateurs risked their own safety to crawl into dangerous ruins when they heard cries for help. There were some dramatic rescues, but just as many sad stories when injured people could not be reached in time.

There was nothing for it but to perform a double amputation.

Acts of bravery were common. One momentous act took place in the ruins of the Pyne Gould Corporation building, where a man had been pinned by his legs beneath a concrete column and part of a collapsed floor. The man was bleeding to death as his life lay in the hands of two civilian doctors, a firefighter and a policeman. There was nothing for it but to perform a double amputation. All the rescue team had at their disposal were a hacksaw and a penknife, although the man was able to be anaesthetised with morphine and ketamine. To limit the further loss of blood, tourniquets were tied to both legs. Then time stood still as the crude operation took place. The doctor performing the operation ran out of puff and the policeman, second doctor and the firefighter helped out until the amputation was complete. The freed man was then rushed to an ambulance. He survived because of an extraordinary display of courage by his rescuers, whose grisly task was made even more difficult by a series of aftershocks that threatened to destabilise the area.

A cursory glance at the collapsed and burning CTV building suggested that survivors would be few. However, a group of policemen detected signs of life after climbing onto the roof. They were obliged to attempt several rescues amongst the rubble of the building's lift tower. The latter provided a hazardous setting for with each aftershock more of the tower collapsed. Despite fears for their own safety, the policemen were initially able to rescue a woman and two children. Beyond that, they had to rely on tapping sounds and voices to guide them to at least eight further survivors. Their most courageous act came when, on hearing a woman call for help in the area of the building that was burning, they attempted to reach her with wet clothing draped around their heads as a deterrent to the heat and smoke. They were driven back, but fate dealt them a fair hand. There was a brief change in wind direction, easing the fire hazard, and they were able to clamber down inside the building and pull the woman free.

There were further heroic tales of rescue as the post-quake hours ticked away and horrendous aftershocks, some nearly as sharp as the original quake, continued to cause anxiety. Being extricated from the rubble was one thing, but the business of being rescued from tall buildings after stairwells had been wiped out brought its own potential perils. In the Forsyth Barr building, people were trapped between the 15th and 17th floors. They could talk about getting up to the roof and hoping helicopters would lift them clear, but there was always the possibility of the building collapsing further. The group that gathered on the 17th floor sought a more expeditious exit.

Eventually the problem was solved. A crane could be seen winching survivors out of the lower floor windows in a large basket attached to the crane arm. Between the 15th floor and the lower floors, the collapsed stairwells had created a no-go zone. The sight of the crane and its basket must have been encouraging to those trapped on the 17th floor, but somehow it seemed a false hope. The crane didn't appear to have the size and range to reach those waiting on the balconies higher up. Then the crane extended its arm and suddenly the basket was brushing up against the balcony on the 17th floor. All of those that had been trapped were rescued.

The sight of the crane and its basket must have been encouraging to those trapped on the 17th floor.

Personal stories began circulating as the hours passed. One woman needed to get to an outlying suburb some distance away, but her car had been crushed. Public transport obviously wasn't running and she needed to get home to check on the safety of family members.

Overwhelmed by the events of the day and the apparent impossibility of returning home, she sat with her head in her hands on a park bench. A young man on a bicycle stopped to comfort her. When he learned of her predicament he offered the woman his bike. She could get home on that, if she took it carefully. The young man lived only 2 km away and said he would walk home. The woman, in a bit of a fog, accepted his offer and cycled off towards the east. At no point in the exchange was the matter of returning the bike even broached. Who cared about the fate of a bike with all the human misery unfolding?

One unexpected result of her ride home was the need to negotiate the liquefaction in some areas. Liquefaction had become a striking feature of the September quake and was now making its presence felt again. Eastern regions of the city had been built on what had been an extensive swamp. Saturated layers of sand and silt beneath the suburbs were converted into sludge when shaken by the quakes, and the resulting liquefaction was forced to the surface where it clogged streets and ruined property foundations.

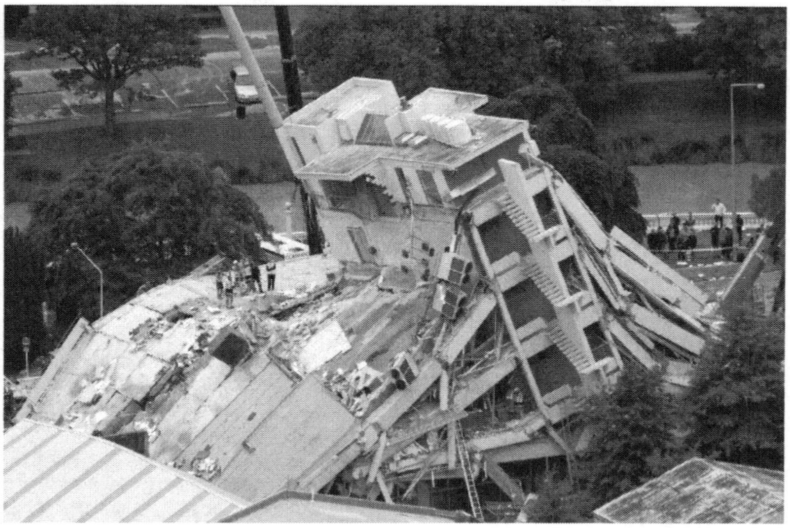

When the Pyne Gould Corporation building collapsed, it killed 18 people. (Otago Daily Times)

Many suburbs were badly affected by the quake. It wasn't just the liquefaction. A large number of houses had been damaged in such a way that they were uninhabitable. Foundations were cracked and buckled. One of the blessings of the quake was that few residents living in the suburbs suffered serious injury. However, thousands of properties were later earmarked for demolition. It became common to hear residents describe their ruined properties as 'munted', a phrase favoured by younger generations in the wider world but soon to be used extensively by many Christchurch folk.

Christchurch became a wasteland. Some people were drawn to it in the interests of helping. Many locals, traumatised by the destruction and death, were driven away. It was estimated that within weeks of the event something like 70,000 Cantabrians left the city because of houses that were no longer safe or habitable. Others left because of the dislocation caused by damaged infrastructure. Basic services like water supply and sewerage were severed, and a persistent image of the post-quake period was of the port-a-loo toilet. They appeared everywhere in ruined suburbs.

Then there were the incessant aftershocks. They drove even more Christchurch people away, either permanently or on a temporary basis. The city of Timaru in South Canterbury experienced an increase in population of close to 20 per cent. Other towns and cities welcomed many refugees from the devastated Christchurch hinterland, where it was estimated that several thousand houses would have to be demolished. More than that, it was considered likely that some areas of the suburbs would never be reoccupied because of the instability of the land.

Those who stayed were faced with some daunting facts. Although power was restored to 75 per cent of the city within three days, it was estimated that water supplies and functional sewage systems would take several years to restore in areas badly affected by liquefaction.

In many ways the Christchurch earthquake was also a modern global disaster. King's Education School was located within the portals of the collapsed CTV building. The school taught the English language to a wide range of nationalities. Twenty-eight Japanese, 23 Chinese and students from 14 other national groups lost their lives there. New Zealand became inextricably linked to many foreign countries and their grieving inhabitants. Christchurch might have been our disaster, but with 65 foreigners losing their lives, it was theirs too.

It was heartening to see the assistance given to the city by Australians who, in a reciprocal gesture prompted by New Zealand's help after the deadly bushfires had struck Victoria in 2009, crossed the Tasman in significant numbers. The Japanese, who would suffer their own quake and tsunami less than a month after the Christchurch event, later provided help too in another reciprocal act.

In 2015 Christchurch is rising from the ashes. The city is in recovery mode and many of its citizens are returning. Some of it may be symbolic. The Transitional Cathedral, commonly known as the 'Cardboard Cathedral', was built of cardboard tubes, timber and steel, with a roof of polycarbon, and was the first significant building opened as part of the Christchurch rebuild. And the shopping mall made out of shipping containers in Cashel Street called Re:START has seen people return to the central city. Tales of deprivation continue to emerge, but so do the stories of human kindness and heroics. People are beginning to think positively about the new Christchurch that is emerging. If Napier could rise from the ashes after the 1931 quake to become the art deco capital of New Zealand, who can say what Christchurch might become?

31

SKY HIGH

The Carterton air balloon tragedy 2012

From the late 1970s adventure activities started gaining popularity throughout New Zealand, rapidly growing into a recognised industry of its own. White-water rafting quickly took hold, proving especially popular with an older clientele, who might have realised they had spent too much time pursuing safe, well-chaperoned activities in their youth, and were ready to do something probably quite safe but with a tantalising hint of danger. White-water rafting spawned black water rafting, then people were parachuting, skydiving, para-skiing or para-ponting unde the supervision of trained guides or taking wicked jetboat rides through impossible narrow gaps in jagged rocks.

Then, in the mid-1980s, a New Zealander, A. J. Hackett, plunged off the Eiffel Tower on a bungy cord into the arms of a waiting gendarme. The incident attracted worldwide attention and soon bungy-jumping became a viable commercial enterprise in New Zealand. Before long tourists were flocking to the country, travelling to all parts looking for the latest adventure thrill.

Hot-air ballooning became popular, not so much as a thrill activity but as something completely safe and serene. But it looked dangerous, with a huge naked flame licking into an elliptical sphere of super-heated air contained only by walls of thin, supposedly fire-resistant fabric. The pastime also appeared to be dependent on little or no wind, the entire concept surely prone to some random gust. We did hear of hot-air ballooning accidents, for example when two hot-air balloons collided over Alice Springs in 1989, and in Canterbury two tourists drowned when a hot-air balloon was blown out to sea in 1995. But generally the activity proved to be safe, and commercial operators were able to quote impressive safety statistics.

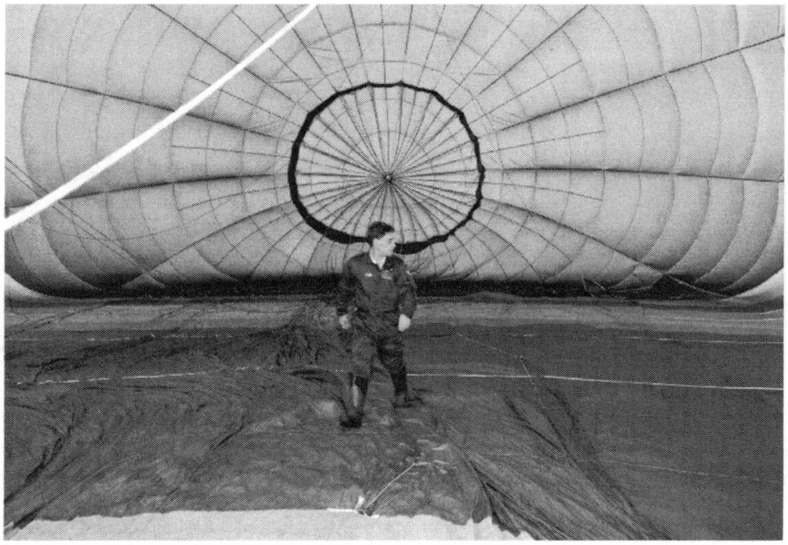

Lance Hopping inflates the hot air balloon in readiness for flight.
(Geoff Walker Photographer, Masterton)

Known for its funnelling southerlies, the Wairarapa would not seem an ideal place for ballooning, but there were sufficient calm days to make passenger flights commercially viable. In 1990 Lance Hopping, owner of Ballooning New Zealand Ltd, set up an operation in Carterton in conjunction with Early Morning Balloons Ltd. Hopping was well-known in ballooning circles and was safety officer for the iconic Balloons over Wairarapa festival. He had accumulated more than 1000 hours piloting balloons in the Carterton area over 15 years. He was known as a 'top bloke' in the community where he worked part-time as a truancy officer, bringing him into regular contact with families whose children had, for one reason or another, ended up on the wrong side of the tracks. But he was also involved with the Seven Day Club, a local bikers' bar, where passing a joint of cannabis was as common as a handshake. His friends later said they usually observed Hopping declining such offers.

The balloon rides tended to be busy over the summer months and, in keeping with industry trends, had come to include add-ons like perfect coffee appearing at just the right moment, a cooked breakfast ready and waiting, and beaming photographs taken at that never-to-berepeated moment. In the days leading up to the disaster, the owner had indicated he wished to resume control of the balloon to build up his own business, and Hopping had been involved in discussions about obtaining a replacement balloon the night before the accident.

On the morning of 7 January 2012, Hopping was up and about well before 6a.m. and released a sensor balloon which transmitted data used to determine likely winds. Satisfied with this, Hopping contacted his ground crew by text and met his customers on site by 6.12a.m., the excited passengers assisting to roll out and inflate the enormous balloon as part of a well-rehearsed build-up. Ten people, mostly couples, were waiting to climb aboard, two having been given the ride as a birthday gift.

After a safety briefing, lift-off took place at 6.43a.m. into a clear blue Wairarapa sky. The balloon made a wide traverse over the township, then circled to the north-west of Carterton where Hopping radioed his ground crew that he was looking at an area near Somerset Road as a suitable landing site, having landed in that area several times before. The ground crew then headed to Somerset Road by utility truck, followed by relatives who had come to share the excitement with those on board. Everyone was taking photographs.

He was known as a 'top bloke' in the community where he worked part-time as a truancy officer.

At 7.15a.m. the balloon was swooping low towards Somerset Road over a silage paddock fringed on two sides with power lines. An irrigation system was also in operation there. For those reasons it did not seem likely the balloon would land there, and the ground crew radioed Hopping asking whether he had seen an untethered horse in the paddock beyond, and he confirmed that he had. Expecting the balloon to try for the horse paddock, the ground crew were looking for gates when they became aware the burners were suddenly full on, then heard Hopping yelling out for everyone to get down. *Looking up, they saw the balloon had drifted towards high tension lines.*

Looking up, they saw the balloon had drifted towards high tension lines on one side of the silage paddock and was trying to climb above the wires when the passenger basket snagged. Being reassured they would not be electrocuted, some passengers were trying to unsnag the wires with their bare hands while the burners tried to lift the basket free. But instead the basket was sliding menacingly towards a power pole, where an 11,000-volt short circuit ignited the gas supply and the basket. Two terrified passengers jumped 60 feet to the ground, where they both died from their injuries.

Meanwhile the intense heat was sufficient to completely melt one of the wires, freeing the basket which immediately rose to 350 feet, by which time the flames had engulfed the entire balloon. Everything fell to the ground. With 11 deaths in hideous circumstances, it was New Zealand's worst aviation disaster since the Erebus crash of 1979. Those who witnessed the scene or heard the screams of the victims, including the watching families, were traumatised and experienced nightmares for months. Three volunteer firemen were so overcome they quit the Fire Service. The shocking news circulated the globe within hours.

Apart from some minor deficiencies in paperwork, the accident enquiry determined the balloon itself was free from defects, attention instead focusing on a measurable quantity of tetrahydrocannibol in the pilot's blood and urine samples. One or two people gave evidence that they had seen the pilot smoking something that could have been a joint on a balcony minutes before the flight, and the blood samples were consistent with a recent inhalation. Friends of the pilot were sure he was too good a bloke to be so reckless as to fly under the influence of drugs, but admitted they knew he smoked cannabis regularly.

Some people made statements to police but would not testify at the enquiry. Evidence emerged that earlier flights had been cancelled because Hopping was 'too pissed', and on another occasion people had observed that he clearly needed assistance to carry out basic physical tasks. A fellow balloonist stated that the two who jumped exacerbated matters, having been briefed to stay with the basket in any emergency. He said it was their fault the balloon climbed suddenly instead of being allowed to ground while the fire was extinguished. When wreckage was examined, the extinguisher was already empty.

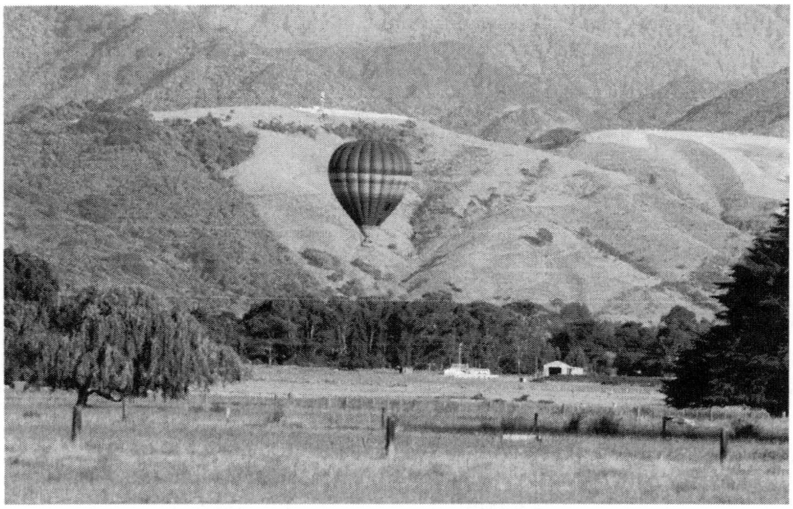

Seconds from disaster – the balloon in the last stages of its final descent. (Geoff Walker Photographer, Masterton)

The disaster sparked an outrage, many people convincing themselves the Civil Aviation Administration were to blame. It was found that Hopping's medical certificate had expired six weeks beforehand and he was thus flying without a licence. People asked why the Minister of Transport did not have a system in place where such people were forcibly stopped. Surely his medical examiner was at fault for not detecting his use of drugs and for accepting Hopping's medical statement at face value.

Nobody seemed to take into account the fact that Hopping himself had already breached the Civil Aviation Act by signing his medical declaration without disclosing his use of cannabis, however infrequent. Such a breach in itself attracted a prison term. At the same time, it seemed inexplicable that a serious complaint concerning Hopping's binge-drinking habits and use of cannabis, made by a member of the public to Civil Aviation some years earlier, had resulted in no prosecution. CAA weakly pointed out that it did not believe it had sufficient evidence to discharge its onus of proof, so no further action was taken. Families of the victims were unanimous in their conviction that they would never have allowed their loved ones to take the flight had they known.

Many photographs of the disaster given to police were subject to a restraining order to prevent media publication. Early Morning Balloons had an arrangement with local photographer Geoff Walker to take pictures for later sale to the participants. For humanitarian and also copyright reasons, Walker supported the move to disallow public reproduction of his shots, some of which were horrific. When in October 2014 a coroner ruled that four photographs could be made public, Walker appealed, but his appeal was opposed not only by TVNZ but also by the families of the victims. In January 2015 Mr Walker withdrew his objection to the release of the four photographs, renewing media attention on the disaster.

Investigators were a little puzzled by the low pass over the silage paddock, where the same paddock had been crossed minutes earlier at a safe height. Unconfirmed information came to light that sometimes Hopping's flights would finish with a low swoop over the ground, one allegedly so low that the basket splashed through a river. Perhaps the low pass over the silage paddock was intended as some sort of thrill to end the flight. If so, this was clearly hazardous in the presence of high-tension wires.

Investigators pointed out it would have been possible to ground the balloon in the paddock, which would have spared everybody. Just what was going through Hopping's mind at that moment or what his intentions were, nobody will ever know, but the post-mortem information does give a vital clue. Perhaps a random gust of wind did strike at the just the wrong moment, demanding immediate action by a clear mind in a situation where a slowed reaction time could lead to catastrophe.

Bibliography

Books

Conly, Geoff and Stewart, Graham, *New Zealand Tragedies on the Track.* Grantham House, Wellington, 1986.

Grayland, Eugene C., New Zealand Disasters. A.H. amp; A.W. Reed, Wellington, 1957. Grayland, Eugene, *More New Zealand Disasters.* A.H. & A.W. Reed, Wellington, 1978.

Holmes, Paul, *Daughters of Erebus.* Hodder Moa, Auckland, 2011.

Hunt, Graeme, Scandal at Cave Creek. Waddington Publications in association with the *National Business Review,* Auckland, 1996.

Hutchins, Graham, *Highwater: Floods in New Zealand.* Grantham House, Wellington, 2006.

King, John, *New Zealand Tragedies: Aviation Accidents and Disasters.* Grantham House, Wellington, 1995.

MacFie, Rebecca, *Tragedy at Pike River.* Awa Press, Wellington, 2013.

McCloy, Nicola, *New Zealand Disasters.* Whitcoulls, Auckland, 2004.

Monigatti, Rex, *New Zealand Sensations.* A.H. & A.W. Reed, Wellington, 1962.

Morris, Bruce, *The Country's Darkest Days.* Wilson & Horton, Auckland, 1981.

Parham, W.T., *Island Volcano.* William Collins (NZ), Auckland, 1973.

Stewart, Graham, *Tangiwai: A Christmas Eve Tragedy.* Grantham House, Wellington, 2013.

Vette, Gordon, *Impact Erebus.* Hodder and Stoughton, Auckland, 1983.

Magazines and newspapers

Dominion

New Zealand Herald

New Zealand Memories

New Zealand Wings

Sunday Star Times

Taranaki Daily News

Waikato Times

Websites

www.aviationarcheology.com

www.bellblock.co.nz

www.christchurchnz.com

www.en.wikipedia.org

www.familytreecircles.com

www.freepages.genealogy.rootsweb.ancestry.com

www.hillaryoutdoors.co.nz

www.hwe.niwa.co.nz

www.info.geonet.org.nz

www.ketehamilton.peoplesnetworknz.info

www.my.christchurchcitylibraries.com

www.newswire.co.nz

www.nzetc.victoria.ac.nz

www.nzherald.co.nz

www.nzhistory.net.nz

www.nzterritory.com

www.odt.co.nz

www.paperspast.govt.nz

www.radionz.co.nz

www.rnzafproboards.com

www.ruralfirehistory.org.nz

www.scoop.co.nz

www.stats.govt.nz

www.stuff.co.nz

www.tauranga.kete.net.nz

www.teara.govt.nz

www.theatreview.org.nz

www.theprow.org.nz

Other research sources

Aircraft Accident Report 85–006, Civil Aviation Administration, Wellington, 1985.

Aircraft Accident Report 85–015, Civil Aviation Administration, Wellington, 1985.

Aircraft Accident Report 96–006, Civil Aviation Administration, Wellington, 1996.

Attwood, Steve, 'The untold story', *Sunday Star-Times,* 28 April 1996.

Commission of Inquiry into the Collapse of a Viewing Platform at Cave Creek near Punakaiki on the West Coast 1995, Department of Internal Affairs, Wellington.

'Lessons from SFA', *New Zealand Wings Magazine,* August 1997.

New Zealand Archives: RNZAF, Mustangs, New Zealand 2404 & 2411.

Report of the Royal Commission on the Pike River Coal Mine Tragedy, New Zealand Government, Wellington, 2012.

Report of the Royal Commission to Inquire into the Crash on Mt Erebus, Antarctica of a DC 10 Aircraft operated by Air New Zealand Ltd, New Zealand Government, Wellington, 1981.

Report to Trustees of the Sir Edmund Hillary Outdoor Pursuit Centre of New Zealand. Mangatepopo Gorge Incident, 15 April 2008. Brookes, Wellington, 2009.

Speden, Graeme, 'Construction of a disaster', *Dominion,* 23 November 1995.

TAIC Aviation Inquiry 12–001, Wellington, 2013.

Taranaki Daily News archive, December 1953.

Thompson, Wayne, 'Cave Creek Haunts Survivor', *New Zealand Herald,* 18 March 2005.

Front Cover Flap

A full train plunges into a raging river at Tangiwai; the Wahine is tossed onto rocks at the entrance to Wellington Harbour; an Air New Zealand DC10 plunges into Mt Erebus; an earthquake destroys Christchurch ... disasters like these are known to all New Zealanders: they are part of our history, part of our lives. But New Zealand has experienced many more disasters—incidents less well known, but shocking, surprising, brutal, bizarre.

Graham Hutchins and Russell Young describe some of the most extraordinary events in New Zealand history. Who knew that a fire killed 39 people at Seacliff Mental Hospital in 1942? That 10 people died in a lahar on White Island in 1914? That a yacht race between Lyttelton and Wellington in 1951 resulted in 10 fatalities? That a tornado ripped through 150 houses in Hamilton in 1948? A fire raging through Raetihi in 1918 was so fierce it destroyed houses, shops and 11 timber mills. Drownings were so common here in the 19th century that they were called 'the New Zealand death'.

These and many other remarkable stories are told in this truly eye-opening book. While it describes accidents and tragedies, it also reveals acts of heroism and valour. For when vulnerable human beings make mistakes, others often achieve superhuman feats of rescue and daring. Some of the stories in this book show that we underestimate Mother Nature at our peril, but many also testify to the courage of the human spirit. Few books are genuine page-turners; this one is.

Back Cover Flap

Graham Hutchins **has been writing books for over thirty years. Most of these have been non-fiction, covering such subjects as rugby, cricket, popular music and railways. Among his best-selling books published by Exisle are *Stop the Train! I want to get on, Great New Zealand Railway Journeys, Last Train to Paradise* and *Eight Days a Week.* Graham and his wife live in Hamilton. He and his co-author Russell Young have been close friends since the age of five.**

Russell Young **graduated from the University of Auckland and worked in Te Kuiti for 30 years before moving to Marlborough in 2004, where he combines business with a passion for flying. He gained his private pilot licence at the age of 23, and nine years ago acquired a Piper Cherokee 180. In 2013 he published *The Story of Te Kuiti.* Russell and his wife live in Blenheim.**

Back Cover Material

Thirty-one devastating events that changed New Zealand.
Thirty-one enthralling stories that every New Zealander should know.

***

This book hobours those who lost their lives and salutes the heroic deeds of the selfless rescuers.

A

B

C

G

H

S

T

Y

Z

Printed in Dunstable, United Kingdom

91336858R00208